10/06 $15.00

Volume 5
Recognizing Your Emotions

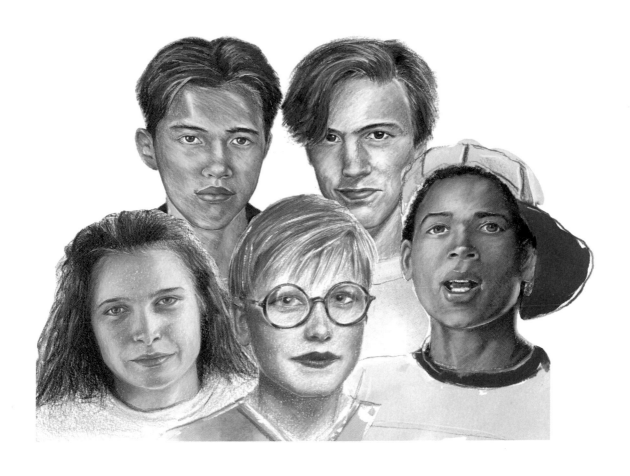

World Book, Inc.
a Scott Fetzer company
Chicago

Staff

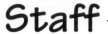

President
Robert C. Martin

Vice President, Publisher
Michael Ross

Editorial

Managing Editor
Maureen Mostyn Liebenson

Contributing Editor
Jeanne Johnson

Permissions Editor
Janet T. Peterson

Art

Executive Director
Roberta Dimmer

Art Director
Wilma Stevens

Designer
John Horvath

Photography Director
Sandra Dyrlund

Photographs Editor
Carol Parden

Production Assistant
John Whitney

Cover Design
Carol Gildar

Research

Executive Director, Product Development and Research Services
Paul A. Kobasa

Research Manager
Loranne Shields

Researcher
Juliet Martinez

Production

Director, Pre-Press and Manufacturing
Carma Fazio

Manufacturing Manager
Steve Hueppchen

Senior Production Manager
Madelyn Underwood

Proofreader
Anne Dillon

For information on other World Book publications, visit our Web site at http://www.worldbook.com or call: 1-800-WORLDBK (967-5325). For information about sales to schools and libraries call: 1-800-975-3250 (United States) or 1-800-837-5365 (Canada).

World Book, Inc.
233 North Michigan Avenue
Chicago, IL 60601

Library of Congress Cataloging-in-Publication Data

World Book's managing your teenage life.
    p. cm.
  Rev. ed. of: Growing up: a handbook to becoming an adult. c1993.
  Includes bibliographical references and index.
  Contents: v. 1. Staying in shape—v. 2. Looking your best—v. 3. Eating for health—v. 4. Understanding sexuality—v. 5. Recognizing your emotions.
  ISBN 0-7166-6700-2 (set)—ISBN 0-7166-6701-0 (v. 1)—ISBN 0-7166-6702-9 (v. 2)—
ISBN 0-7166-6703-7 (v. 3)—ISBN 0-7166-6704-5 (v. 4)—ISBN 0-7166-6705-3 (v. 5)
  1. Teenagers—Health and hygiene—Juvenile literature. 2. Adolescence—Juvenile literature.
  3. Teenagers—Psychology—Juvenile literature. 4. Adolescent medicine—Juvenile literature.
  [1. Teenagers—Health and hygiene. 2. Teenagers—Psychology. 3. Life skills.] I. World Book, Inc. II. Growing up. III. Title: Managing your teenage life.

RA777.G76 2003
613'.0433—dc21   2002024984

Printed in Singapore

1 2 3 4 5 6 06 05 04 03 02

Medical Consultants

Medical Editor
Erich E. Brueschke, M.D., F.A.A.F.P.
Vice Dean of Rush Medical College,
   Professor and Chairman of Family
   Medicine, and Senior Attending
   Physician
Rush-Presbyterian-St. Luke's Medical
   Center

Associate Medical Editors
Susan Vanderberg-Dent, M.D.
Associate Professor, Program
   Director of Rush-Illinois
   Masonic Family Practice Residency,
   and Associate Attending Physician
Rush-Presbyterian-St. Luke's Medical
   Center

Frances Bryan Brueschke, R.N.
Consultant in Family Medicine
   Nursing
Department of Family Medicine
Rush-Presbyterian-St. Luke's Medical
   Center

Steven K. Rothschild, M.D.
Assistant Professor, Assistant
   Chairman for Clinical Programs in
   Family Medicine, and Associate
   Attending Physician
Rush-Presbyterian-St. Luke's Medical
   Center

Diane D. Homan, M.D.
Assistant Professor of Family Medicine
   and Assistant Attending Physician
Rush-Presbyterian-St. Luke's Medical
   Center

Assistant Medical Editors
Maureen A. Murtaugh, Ph.D., R.D.
Assistant Professor
Department of Clinical Nutrition
Rush University, College of Health
   Sciences

Linda O. Douglas, M.D.
Assistant Professor of Family Medicine
Rush-Presbyterian-St. Luke's Medical
   Center

Sex Education Consultant
Beverly K. Biehr, M.S., M.A., C.F.L.E.
Facilitator, Family Life/AIDS Education
   Program
Chicago Public Schools

CONTENTS

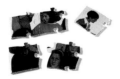

Changing lives

During your exciting journey into young adulthood, your life will change in many ways. As your body matures, you'll experience new emotions. You may begin to question attitudes and situations that you previously accepted. You'll view yourself and others differently. Adolescence is an exhilarating, but sometimes overwhelming, time. Growing up is learning to make choices – choices about your life style, about your friends, about yourself. You'll want to make your own decisions about your life rather than accept other people's choices for you. You may even want to reorganize the pieces of the great jigsaw puzzle of your life in your own way.

An important thing to remember is that *everybody* goes through these changes. You're not alone. Everyone grows up. Every adult was once an adolescent.

Who is grown up?

Your body begins to change into an adult's body when its inner rhythms tell it to. This time of change is called puberty. During puberty, your body becomes physically able to bear or father a child. But most people are not emotionally ready to be parents until many years later. At what age do you become a young adult mentally?

The answer depends on many things. One important factor is your position in the family. You may be the oldest child and used to leading others. Perhaps you feel more grown up than other people your age. If you're a middle child in your family, you may be torn between wanting more responsibility and wanting to hold back. If you're the youngest, you'll have learned from older brothers and sisters, so you may be quite mature for your age. On the other hand, your family may still see you as the "baby" and not want you to grow up too fast. There's no one age when everyone may be said to be grown up. Like everyone else, you'll grow up at your own pace.

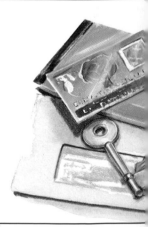

IN THE EYES OF THE LAW
When does the law say you are a young adult and not a child? A person legally becomes an adult at 18 in most states of the United States, in most Canadian provinces, and in most European countries. At 18 you can vote, serve in your country's military without your parents' consent, and sign contracts.

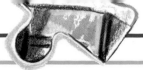

Reading through

Recognizing Your Emotions will help you understand how your feelings will change as you grow up and how you can prepare for those changes. It is divided into four sections. Each one deals with a piece of the great puzzle of life. The first section looks at you as an individual. It will help you find out more about yourself. You may think you know yourself quite well already. But it's important that you get to know and like yourself as much as possible. It's also important to be proud of yourself and to know your potential. Many young people question the rules set by their families and by society. You'll find suggestions in this book about how to deal with questions and problems that might arise.

The second section discusses your family and the way your relationship with them changes as you grow up. When you're very young, your family is probably the most important influence in your life. But as you get older, your ideas may change. Things you accepted when you were a child may become issues you want to challenge when you are an adolescent. Life isn't always smooth; everyone has problems to overcome. So parts of this section are specifically written to help you deal with them. One part focuses on parent separation and divorce. Another involves death and grief. Sooner or later, everyone must face a loss, so it's good to know what can happen and how you might feel.

The third section concerns friends and how you relate to them. Naturally, your friends are very important to you. Some friendships you make when you're a teen-ager may last the rest of your life. In this book, you can read about different types of friendship. As you reach puberty, you begin to discover that you have sexual feelings as well as emotional feelings. So there are pages to help you deal with boyfriends and girlfriends, love, and sexual relationships. You'll also read about peer pressure. Other pages give you the facts on alcohol, tobacco, and drug abuse.

The last section discusses many of the new emotions you might feel as you grow up. You may, for instance, find that you've become very moody – happy one moment and sad the next. You can find out in this section how to handle these moods and how to learn from your experiences. You'll also find out how to recognize feelings of uncertainty, anger, jealousy, depression, and boredom, and how to cope with them. For example, you may be experiencing stress because of exams at school. How do you cope? Perhaps you're shy or lonely, or sometimes just need a little more confidence. This section will show you how to give yourself that boost. The last part of this section looks at your role in the community and your feelings about being an adult in the big, wide, exciting world.

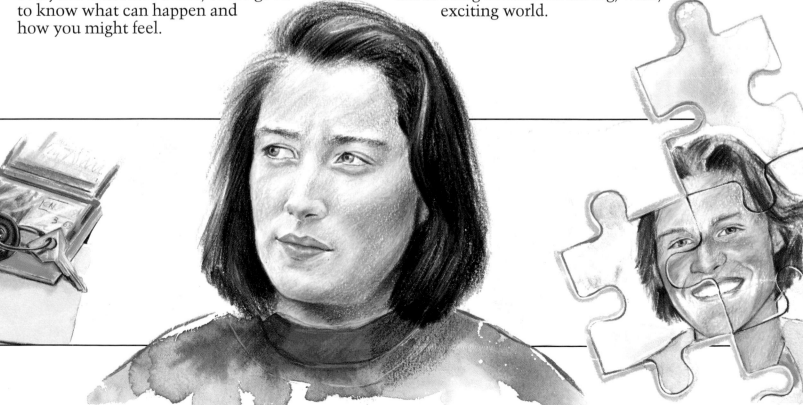

Who am I?

When you're a teen-ager, not only does your body change, but your thoughts and feelings change as well. You experience new emotions that influence how you see yourself and others. At times, you might feel you just want to rewrite the rulebook on how to live with the world, your family, your friends, and, especially, yourself.

Some people find that adolescence is a time of tremendous ups and downs. Your mood can swing from ecstasy to gloom in the space of a single morning. (As you'll find out, your hormones can be partly responsible for these mood swings.) You may find you keep changing your mind as well. One day you'll be quite sure about something, and the next day you'll wonder how you could ever have thought that way.

Whatever happens, it's important that you stay positive about yourself. Remember that each new day makes you a little older, and, more important, each new experience can make you a little wiser.

All in the family

When you're a child, people like to tell you how much you resemble some other member of your family. You're told that you have your mother's eyes, your father's ears, or your grandmother's nose. People will continue to make these kinds of comparisons as you get older. Yet no two people have exactly the same combination of features and feelings. Of course, you have inherited physical traits and learned mannerisms from your parents, but you're an individual and a unique person.

You're also now an adolescent, and adolescence is the time for you to define yourself. You can identify the special qualities that make you feel good about yourself. You can also get rid of some of those qualities you don't like.

Influences in your life

All throughout your childhood, your family was probably the most important influence on you.

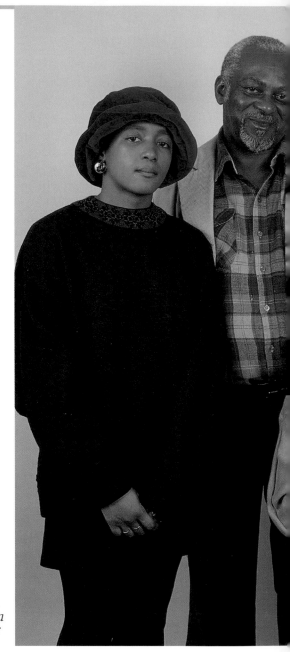

You are both an individual and a member of your family.

You learned from your parents how to behave. You learned how to get along with other people. You learned what was right and what was wrong.

You probably didn't question this influence from your family. You accepted it. It's part of growing up.

But now you have become aware that other

WHAT KIND OF PERSON ARE YOU?

When you're feeling confused about who you are, it might be a good time to ask yourself some questions. For instance:

What do you most like about
     yourself?
What makes you happy?
What pleases you?
What makes you angry?
What excites you?
What bores you?
How do you like to spend your
     free time?

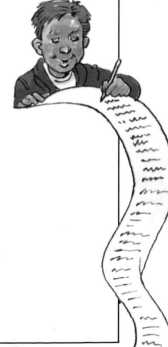

Who are you?

Some questions are more complicated. For instance, a group of friends may be talking about a television show that they all enjoy. Do you agree with them because you genuinely enjoy the program too, or because you don't want to be different? On the other hand, do you disagree just to be contrary or to draw attention to yourself?

Answering these questions honestly can be hard. But finding out what you think helps you learn what's important to you. And knowing yourself helps you let others see the real you.

What do you like?

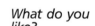

As you grow to know yourself better, you will also discover your limitations. You'll realize that there are some things you cannot do and will never do. Coming to terms with this realization is particularly important. But remember, it's up to you to choose what you want out of life. It's up to you to decide whether you develop your talents and skills. It's up to you to choose which values you take from your family and friends and which values you reject.

people have different ideas. At your age, these people – adults, your friends, people you see and admire on television and in movies – will probably begin to influence the way you think. There's nothing wrong with listening to or even imitating people you admire. But don't forget you have a mind of your own. You need to discover some things for yourself, as well as gather information and ideas from others.

Self-esteem

Self-esteem means knowing and valuing yourself. It means understanding your worth. You have a place in your family and in society. If you were fortunate, you grew up in a home that offered security and support. But if your childhood has been difficult, you may have had to trust your own judgment at an early age rather than rely on your family. In either case, be comfortable with what you are. Self-esteem is *not* conceit. If you have a realistic sense of your own worth, you'll be confident and capable in your own special way.

Self-esteem affects the way you do things, from simple tasks, such as asking for help in a store, to more complicated action, such as dealing with people in authority. It helps you decide what you want out of life and how to work toward achieving it.

Thinking for yourself

There's a difference between taking advice about something and accepting all you are told. If you're not sure about something, it's easy to be influenced by another person's opinion. However, you should listen and then work out your own response. Don't be afraid to question; it shows you are thinking for yourself.

Sticking to your guns

Don't be afraid to say no to people when you mean no. And you don't have to feel guilty about it! Sometimes you may do things you disagree with simply to please others. But part of self-esteem is listening to your inner voice about what's right for you. Be proud to stand up for yourself and your beliefs. Your true friends will admire you for sticking with your decision, and you'll feel happy that you've been true to yourself.

Taking criticism

Your self-esteem can be easily hurt when you are criticized. Try to decide whether you deserve that criticism. Suppose, for example, you're warned at school about not handing your work in on time. You know that it has to be done, but you just don't get around to doing it. Accept that you're at fault and resolve to start doing better.

On the other hand, people may sometimes criticize you unfairly. Perhaps, for example, you couldn't get your work done on time because somebody in your family was ill and you had to spend time looking after them. This kind of criticism is much harder to take. Explain your situation, or you'll feel angry and resentful.

Some criticism is purely spiteful. Occasionally a person in a position of authority will take advantage of that position and criticize someone unfairly. If this happens to you, tell an adult you trust what has happened. You don't have to put up with such criticism.

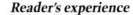

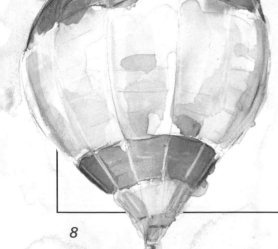

Reader's experience

"My friends all wanted to go up in a hot-air balloon. So when Ben's father arranged it for us, they all got really excited. But I'm scared of heights and knew I couldn't face it. Everyone crowded around me, teasing me and calling me all kinds of names. I felt rotten.

"Then I put my foot down. I said I wasn't going up, and I didn't care what they thought of me. I didn't, either. Everyone stopped giving me a hard time then. I went along on the morning of the flight, and I took some great photographs of the liftoff."
David

Saying what you mean

Sometimes people find it difficult to say what they mean, especially if they're talking about an emotional subject. Maybe they're not clear about what they think, or perhaps they have several ideas at once and don't know which should come first. To say what you mean, you first need to know what you mean. You need to take the time to sort out your thoughts and then rank them in importance to you. That way you begin to get a complete picture of what you want to say and in what order you want to say it. This knowledge will help you feel more confident and build your self-esteem.

Think and speak clearly

When you have something to say, it may get lost if you fail to communicate it properly. Communication skills can be learned. Once you've decided on the most important part of your thought, say it first, then wait for a reaction. Don't repeat yourself. Listen to what others have to say; don't interrupt.

Also, know your audience. Find the right moment to speak out. For example, don't ask a special favor of your parents when you know they are busy. Wait until they have time to listen so they can give you all their attention.

Look people directly in the eye when you're making a point. You're more likely to get your point across. The secret is to be direct and to seem confident.

Your expressions and gestures often mirror the way you feel.

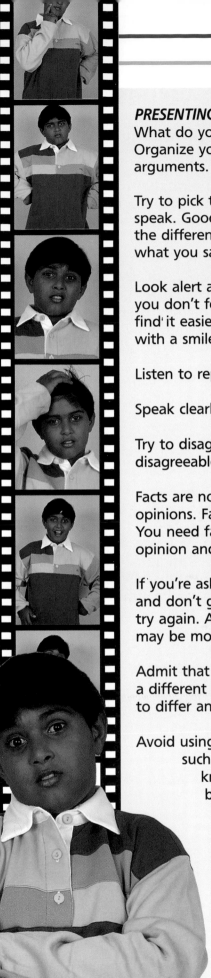

PRESENTING AN OPINION
What do you want to say? Organize your facts and your arguments.

Try to pick the right moment to speak. Good timing can make all the difference in the impact of what you say.

Look alert and pleasant, even if you don't feel that way. You'll find it easier to win people over with a smile.

Listen to replies.

Speak clearly but not loudly.

Try to disagree without being disagreeable.

Facts are not the same as opinions. Facts can be proven. You need facts to back up your opinion and win an argument.

If you're asking for something and don't get it, wait awhile and try again. A different approach may be more successful.

Admit that others have a right to a different point of view. Agree to differ and accept the situation.

Avoid using sweeping statements such as, "Nobody I know has to be home by 8 o'clock at night." Sweeping statements are too easy to disprove.

Use your voice wisely. If you get loud or start whining, you'll seem unsure of yourself.

Working out values

What do you believe in? What do you think is right, and what do you think is wrong? As you grow up, you sort out your own views and opinions, but you also find that others don't necessarily share them. The first disagreements may even come from your own family.

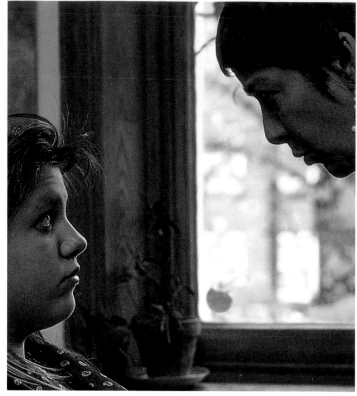

Rebel in the home

As you become a young adult, you may sometimes question your parents' authority, instead of just accepting it. Questioning your parents' values is part of growing up. So far, your parents have been your undisputed guides through life. They have probably tried to pass their values and moral beliefs on to you. But perhaps you're starting to disagree with some of their views.

Perhaps your parents have a certain rule that they feel strongly about. It's usually a waste of time and energy to shout and make a fuss about it. Such behavior often only antagonizes people and makes them more resolved not to budge. If you're really angry, go for a long walk and shout at the trees! Swim some laps, or kick a ball around instead. Exercise helps relieve tension and calm you down.

Many teen-agers question some of their parents' values.

Rebel in society

Every society has rules to govern how people act toward one another. Without rules, we would live in a chaotic world. We all feel more comfortable when we know we can act within certain limits.

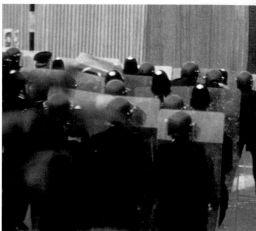

Violent action often causes more problems than it solves.

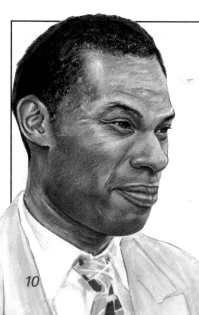

NEGOTIATE
If you disagree with a rule adults have set for you, it's best to keep cool. Remember that your parents have the responsibility as well as the right to set limits for their children. Try to negotiate a new rule with which they are comfortable. You might be able to agree on a trial period. If you follow the rule during that period, you may gain new privileges.

Some rules are written down as laws. It obviously makes sense to have written rules of the road, or drivers would be constantly colliding into each other. In addition, every society has other rules that are unwritten but understood. These are social rules, sometimes called norms. Each of us must decide whether to follow these rules and must understand the potential consequences if we do not.

As you grow older, you may not like everything you see and hear around you. Many people hold very strong opinions about what is right or wrong with the world. You, too, may feel strongly about the way some things are done. You might desperately want to fight for – or against – some change. Working actively to improve your world is admirable and a sign of maturity. But the way you try to change things is important.

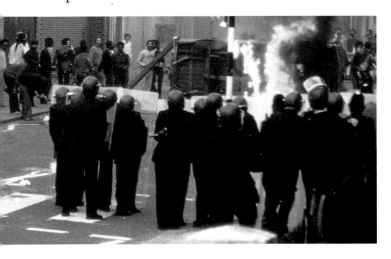

Keep it cool

So you don't agree with something. How do you express your disagreement? Some people turn to violence to change things. But violent talk and violent actions often hurt others and do little to improve the situation. Working peacefully for change in an organized way is generally more effective.

Tolerance is a virtue

In our world of many cultures, races, and religions, we need to tolerate one another's ideas and beliefs.

You can be certain that you'll meet many people in your life who hold beliefs that are different from your own. You'll find some of these people fascinating. With others, you'll "agree to disagree." Some, however, you'll find almost impossible to accept. For example, you may find it just too difficult to hold a polite conversation with a person wearing a fur coat if you're an animal rights activist. You may dislike listening to prejudice of any kind – whether directed at you or in the form of racist or sexist jokes. Unfortunately, you're going to come across intolerance at one time or another. You must decide whether to voice your opinion or walk away without expressing your protest. Remember the rules of good argument from the previous page when you try to voice your opinion, and forget violence. It often feeds on itself and leads to greater injustices.

GROUP ACTION

Individuals can change things in a peaceful way, though change usually doesn't happen overnight. Groups can often bring about change more quickly and successfully. If you feel strongly about an environmental issue, for instance, you'll find many groups to join. Be concerned and informed. Try to decide where you stand on an issue. On the other hand, don't

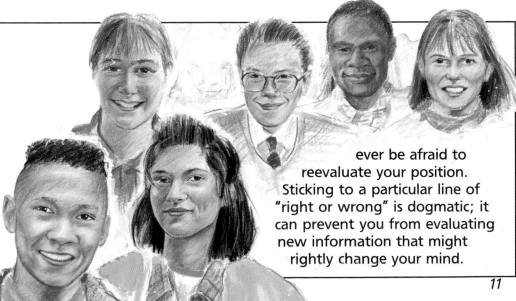

ever be afraid to reevaluate your position. Sticking to a particular line of "right or wrong" is dogmatic; it can prevent you from evaluating new information that might rightly change your mind.

Understand your parents

Believe it or not, your parents can be your best friends, and they may be very pleased that you're growing up. As you mature, relationships within your family will necessarily change. The adults will continue to love and look after you, but the relationship should gradually become one between adults rather than between adult and child.

If you have a problem, try discussing it with one or both of your parents. You may be afraid that they'll be unsympathetic or can't possibly understand, but give them a chance. Ask them how they felt when they were teen-agers. Of course, times were different then, but human nature wasn't. They probably experienced many of the same feelings you're having now. Often what seems important to teen-agers seems minor to adults. By remembering their own adolescence, however, your parents may find it easier to understand how you're feeling.

You may find one parent easier to get along with than the other. Many people do. Some teens get along better with the parent of the same sex, others with the parent of the opposite sex. Everyone's different.

Unfortunately, some parents seem unable to relate to their children. If you feel your parents truly can't understand your problem, talk about it with an adult you trust.

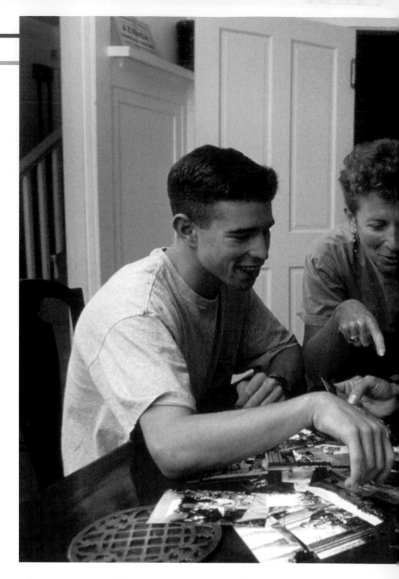

The generation gap

The difference between your personal philosophy and way of life and your parents' is often referred to as the generation gap. Your parents have experienced this gap too – with your grandparents! Whatever your background, the way your parents live and the way you want to live may be different. In fact, seeking your own identity, separate from your parents, is an important part of growing up.

You may think your parents are old. But try to think of them as individuals, not as your mother or father. They have good days and bad days, too. Sometimes parents are under all sorts of pressures. They may worry about money. They may have a difficult or demanding job. They may worry about you or your brothers or sisters. Perhaps an elderly or sick relative in your family needs care. Or perhaps parents are worried about getting old themselves and what that will mean to them and you.

Living with one another

Mother, father, brothers, and sisters – they all can get on one another's nerves from time to time. For example, have you ever objected to your father picking you up from a party because you're afraid your friends might laugh at his clothes? Do you find your mother's loud voice grating? And what about you? Have you ever asked your parents a personal question in a public place? The members of a family can embarrass each other in all sorts of ways, intentionally and unintentionally. But if you try to be sensitive to each other's feelings, and not be too over-sensitive yourself, you'll be less likely to upset each other.

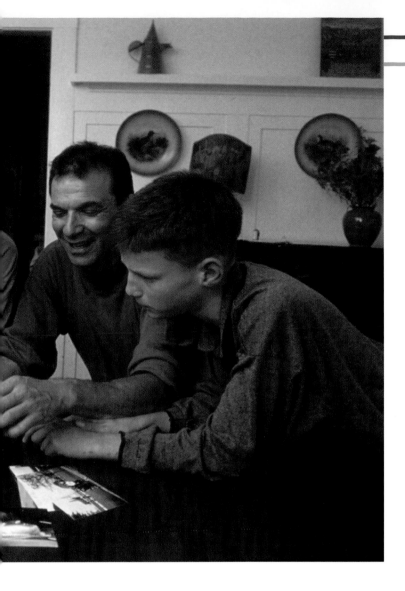

an 11 p.m. curfew for you if they believe other teens your age must be home by 9:30. Help your parents see that your requests aren't extreme. Introduce them to your friends and to your friends' parents. Meeting one another can be an eye-opener – for everyone.

Parents are people, too

Remember, parents can never stop being parents, whatever age they are. Your grandparents may still fuss over your parents. Whatever conflicts you have at home, don't forget that respecting your parents is a sign of maturity. You don't have to agree with everything they believe in, but should respect their views.

Keep in mind, too, that people develop all their lives. This is true of your parents as much as anyone else. As you struggle with the changes that growing up brings, your parents are also adjusting to these changes: your increasing need for privacy, your desire for more freedom, your preference for being with friends rather than family. In addition, parents may be going through changes of their own. A parent who stayed home to raise the family may decide to resume a career. Are you mature enough to cope? You might be called on to share more of the routine responsibilities of running the home. If so, your parents will need to rely on you and trust you more than ever.

Strict parents

Ideally, the rules that exist in your family will protect you while gradually allowing you to take on the responsibilities of being an adult. Yet some rules may seem particularly unfair or harsh. Some adults can be difficult to live with, and you may long for the day when you can leave home and be independent.

Your parents may follow a strict moral code, perhaps as part of their religion. If so, they expect you to observe the same moral code. With strict guidelines, you can at least be clear on the boundaries your parents expect you to respect. Remember, if you want to change things, think before you act. Avoid lying or deceiving your parents, even if honesty seems to bring only arguments. The truth is essential to any meaningful relationship between you and your parents.

Working things out

If you expect your parents to be open and reasonable with you, you owe it to them to be open and reasonable in return. That means telling them where you're going, who you're going with, and what time you'll be back. Think how worried you'd be if your mother and father went out without telling you what they were up to.

What if you want to do something that you think your parents will disapprove of? First of all, determine why you think they'll disapprove. Next, see if you can think of any reasons you should be allowed to do whatever it is, so you have a better chance of persuading your parents. If you treat your parents in a straightforward and honest way, their response is likely to be reasonable. If you antagonize them, you'll make the job harder.

Some parents are anxious about being too permissive. For example, they won't want to set

When parents separate

Divorce is common in the United States and many other countries. Although the parents are the ones who divorce, the pain of divorce affects every member of the family.

Living in a home filled with tension and quarreling is difficult. You may not know what is causing the conflict. You may even think your parents are fighting about you. Your parents may try to "protect" you by pretending nothing is wrong. But this approach may leave you more confused and troubled because you have no way of understanding what is happening. If your parents refuse to discuss their problem openly, you may need to talk to a relative or friend. The uncertainty over whether your parents will stay together or split up can be very hard to cope with.

One reason your parents may find it hard to talk to you is that they themselves don't know what will happen. You may want the fighting — or the silence — to stop and everything to get back to normal. But if your parents decide to separate, you have no choice but to accept their decision.

Feelings about divorce

Many children feel they are to blame when their parents split up. But couples separate because they can't solve problems in their own

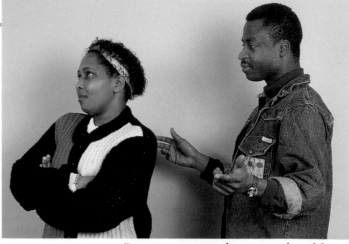

Parents separate because of problems between themselves, not with their children.

relationship, not in their relationship with their children. Parents' problems may include financial difficulties, a poor sexual relationship, or differences in what each one wants out of life. Their problem may not be the fault of either parent — your parents simply may have grown apart. If so, they are unlikely to reconcile, no matter how much you or they wish that could happen. Sometimes children of divorced parents fantasize that their parents will reunite. At first, such fantasies may help you cope. But as time goes on, it's healthier to accept the reality of your parents' separation.

Divorce is usually painful for every member of a family, even if the marriage was unhappy. Divorce brings emotional, financial, and practical changes to a family. It's natural to feel anger and resentment toward parents when they upset the family and your life. You may worry about how a single parent is going to manage your home. You may feel that your parents love you less or wonder how your friends will react to the separation. Remember that all these feelings are a natural response to the turmoil of divorce. And no matter how deep your pain is, it will lessen with time as you learn to accept the situation.

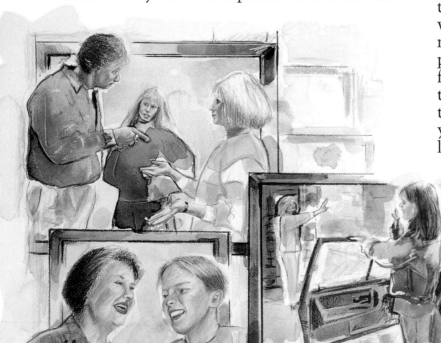

Deciding whom to live with

When people divorce, children usually live with one parent most of the time. Ideally, your parents should take your wishes into account when deciding whom you'll live with. This is an extremely difficult decision for everyone. You may feel that one of your parents needs you more than the other. Perhaps you're afraid that you'll hurt one parent by deciding to live with the other. If you're torn between your parents in this way, you need to be sure that the divorce agreement will allow you to see the absent parent regularly.

The healthiest situation is when parents separate amicably. Neither parent should criticize the other in front of you or pressure you to take sides in their disagreement. If parents' bitterness toward each other persists after their divorce, the pain of the divorce is prolonged for everyone.

When parents remarry

In time, one or both of your parents may get married again. If this happens, you may become part of a new, "blended" family, and you're likely to have mixed feelings. The new marriage may be painful proof that your parents will never reconcile. You may be jealous of your stepparent's special relationship with your father or mother. And if you grow to love your stepparent, you may be afraid that this new marriage will also end in divorce. Or you may think your love is a betrayal of your biological parent.

The relationship between stepparent and stepchild is often different from that between parent and child. You may feel that a stepparent has no right to tell you what to do, for instance. A stepparent who arrives with his or her own children is usually even more difficult to accept. Try to remember that the situation is hard for your new family too. If you can at least tolerate one another, life will be easier.

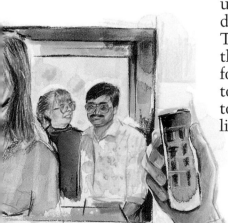

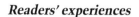

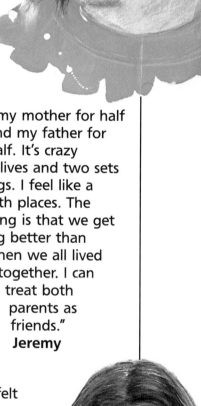

"I live with my mother and my brothers and sisters, and we see my dad on weekends. At first this was really hard. I felt I had to go and see him when I really wanted to be with my friends. I was missing out on all the things they did together. Dad always wanted to take us out for meals and treats, when we just wanted to be with him at home."
Kirsty

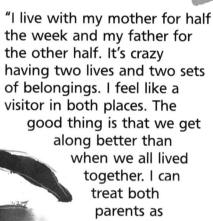

"I live with my mother for half the week and my father for the other half. It's crazy having two lives and two sets of belongings. I feel like a visitor in both places. The good thing is that we get along better than when we all lived together. I can treat both parents as friends."
Jeremy

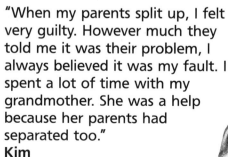

"When my parents split up, I felt very guilty. However much they told me it was their problem, I always believed it was my fault. I spent a lot of time with my grandmother. She was a help because her parents had separated too."
Kim

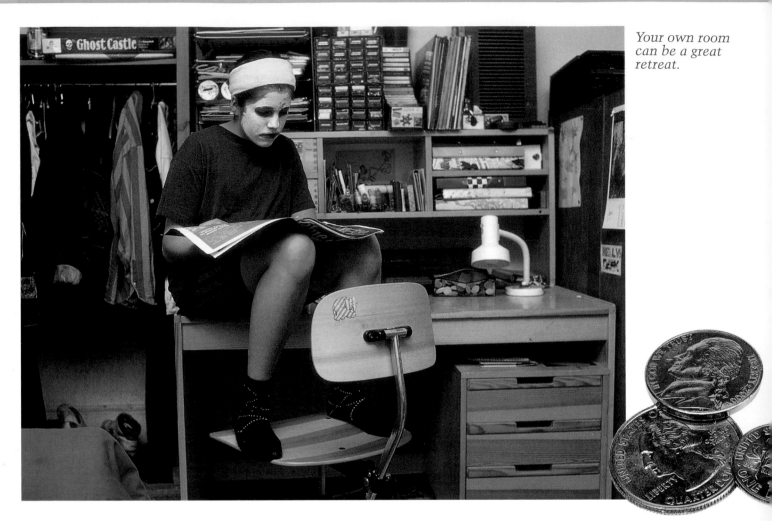

Your own room can be a great retreat.

Standing on your own

At this time of your life, you want your parents to realize you're no longer a child. You want to be treated as an adult. Your parents probably have accepted your growing need to be independent. However, they may not be changing their attitude as quickly as you would like them to. You may have to show them that you can be trusted with more freedom.

At the same time, you may be feeling confused about just how much freedom you want. On one hand, you want to be independent. On the other hand, you want the comfort of being looked after as you have been all your life.

Your own room

While at home, most teen-agers often prefer being alone. If possible, ask for a bedroom of your own. If an entire bedroom is not possible, a room divider or screen can help create a special space for you. Your room can be your retreat, where you can escape from the family and the rest of the world.

Ask your parents if you can decorate your room so that it expresses your personality. However, remember why you wanted your own room in the first place–to have some privacy and be more independent. Having privacy means respecting others' privacy, so don't play your music so loud that it disturbs the rest of the family. And being independent means showing maturity. You are still living in your parents' home, so it's your responsibility to keep your room clean and neat.

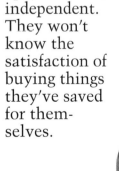

A bank account can make you feel more independent.

Your own money

Do you get spending money from your parents? Some teen-agers manage their allowance so that they can take responsibility for such items as their own clothes, toiletries, and presents. In addition to, or instcad of, an allowance, you may be earning money from a part-time job. If so, saving a little each week is a good idea. Eventually, you'll be able to buy something you really want. Some teens expect their parents will give them money whenever they "need" it. Yet if parents give their kids money every time they overspend or simply want it, the kids may "pay" for it by never becoming financially independent. They won't know the satisfaction of buying things they've saved for themselves.

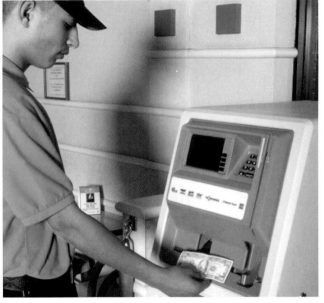

Leaving home

Many people feel ready to leave home when they're in their late teens. They go to college or get a job and want a place of their own. But sometimes the desire to leave home comes too early or for the wrong reason. Have you ever felt like ending an argument by just walking out, slamming the door, and vowing never to come back? Yet, you are likely to want to come back sooner or later, so try not to overreact. Instead, stay and try to work out the problem then and there.

Running away is never glamorous. Teen-age runaways are vulnerable to all kinds of dangers and abuse. Many runaways get involved with drug dealing and even prostitution to support themselves. If you are ever contemplating running away, think carefully. Is there a friend, the parent of a friend, a relative, a social worker, or a teacher you could talk to? Once you've explained your problem, you'll find that people and agencies are ready to help you solve it. Or if by running away you are simply venting your anger with your parents, think again. You can express your anger in a more positive way.

Unfortunately, for a few teen-agers, life at home is truly unbearable. The only solution seems to be to leave home. If they are wise, they'll let someone know they're safe. In the United States, there is a toll-free national runaway switchboard that will pass messages from runaways without revealing their whereabouts. It also offers shelter information and counseling services.

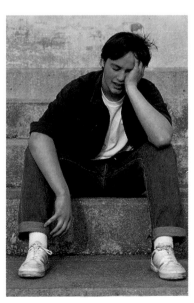

Life on the streets is hard for runaways.

Loss

Everyone's life has times of great sadness as well as happiness. Couples get divorced; loved ones die. You will experience loss in your life, too. You may feel awful when your best friend moves away, or maybe you yourself have moved recently and have had to say goodbye to your friends. At such difficult times, you'll need to understand your unhappiness and come to terms with it.

Death of a pet

The children in some families have grown up all their lives with a family pet that has found a place in everyone's heart. The death of a pet can leave a big hole in your life. It even may be the first death you have experienced. You need to grieve over this death like any other.

Death of a close relative

When somebody close to you dies, you may find yourself in a state of shock. You may feel numb. Sometimes you can't believe the person is gone. You might find yourself expecting him or her to walk into your life again. For some people, this state of mind lasts a few weeks; for others, it goes on a great deal longer. However, eventually you'll be able to pick up the threads of your life and return to normal. If you need to, you can read more on this difficult subject in the article on the opposite page.

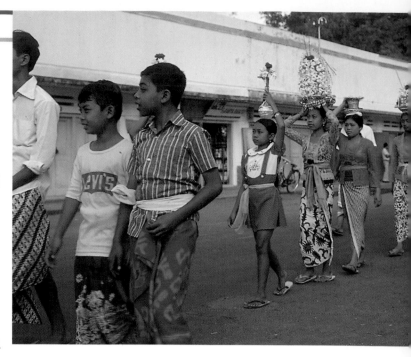

Saying goodbye

In many societies, a funeral takes place when someone has died. This event brings together those who knew the deceased person and helps the grieving process begin. A funeral is a time both to say goodbye and to celebrate the life of the person who has passed away. It also recognizes that those left behind are distressed.

Some adults believe that children should be protected from the details of death. In other families, people are afraid to talk about death at all. This unwillingness to talk about death can cause a problem because it doesn't help the survivors come to terms with it.

Grieving is a normal process that helps relieve the pain of losing something you love. When you experience a sad time like this, it's often comforting to be near your family and close friends. And sharing your feelings about your loss helps the healing process. Remembering the deceased person together will also help you deal openly with the pain you're all experiencing.

Sometimes, friends will be embarrassed in your company. They probably feel upset and sad for you, but they may not know how to talk to you about your loss. Reassure them that you can cope and that you need them around you. Try to keep your school and social life as normal as possible.

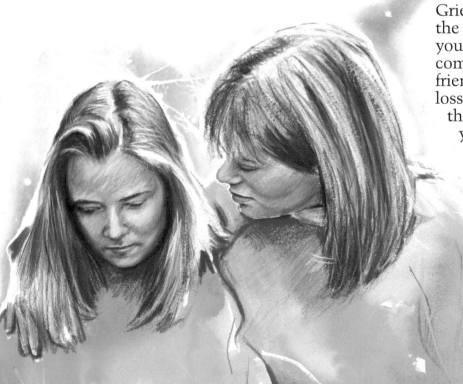

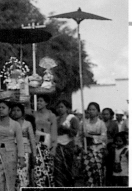

Young people take part in a funeral procession in Indonesia.

A funeral is a solemn occasion.

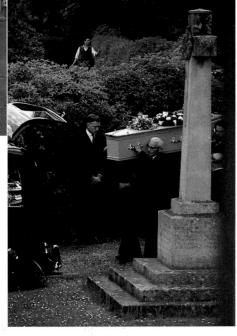

Coping with grief

Throughout our lives, we learn to love people and depend upon them. When a loved one dies, we go through a whole series of emotions to try to make sense of what has happened. Everybody has his or her own way of dealing with grief. Some people need to cry; others need to express anger. Some people need the company and support of friends and family; others need time alone. What's important is that the grieving person be allowed to feel the grief and take as much time as he or she needs to heal.

The first reaction to a death is often shock. Those who are left behind may feel helpless. They sometimes try to deny the death. This feeling may turn to anger because now they are alone – left to fend for themselves. People sometimes feel guilty when someone they love has died. They think back to things they might have done to improve the relationship or make things happen differently. Sometimes, depression takes over. Only as time passes and new experiences take their place among the memories of the lost loved one, does a feeling of acceptance develop.

Because grief is such a strong emotion, it has a physical effect on our bodies. The symptoms of grief may come in waves. There may be feelings of panic as the hormone adrenalin is released in the body. Grief often brings temporary indigestion and heartburn; sleeplessness; a loss of appetite; a feeling of tension in the head; and nervous, irritable behavior. Most people find that crying offers release from tension.

Although it's often difficult to do, keeping busy and active helps people get over their grief. Exercise is particularly helpful because it reduces physical stress.

If you have lost someone you love, you need time and a great deal of understanding to get over it. You may also need to talk to a sympathetic friend. Above all, you must be allowed to grieve and mourn in your own way and in your own time.

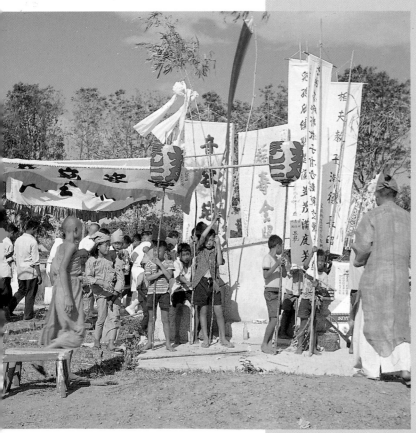

A funeral in Thailand.

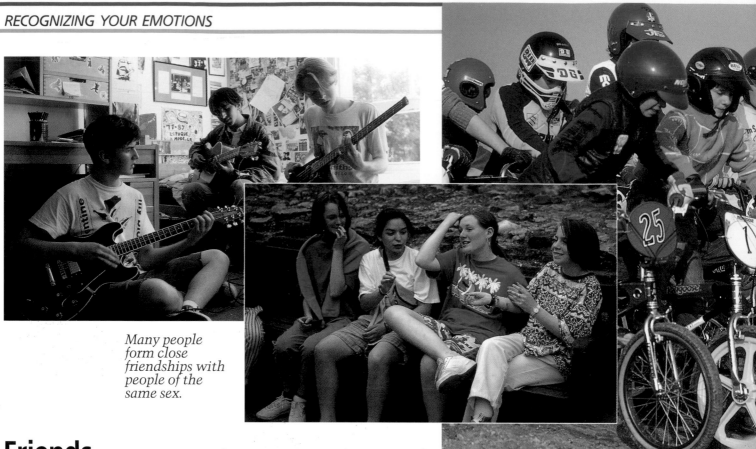

Many people form close friendships with people of the same sex.

Friends

Do you spend a lot of time with your friends? The people you make friends with when you are a teen-ager are very important. You may be friends with some of them for the rest of your life.

Of course, not all your friends are close friends. There are people in your life with whom you are friendly without being special friends. This outer circle of friends is very important, too.

You'll find lots of possible friends in a large group.

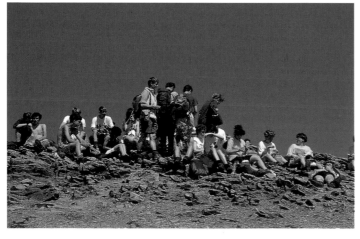

Making friends

If you want friends, you have to make an effort. Sitting shyly in a corner and never saying a word won't work; people will naturally think you don't care about knowing them. Try smiling and saying, "Hi." Get involved with other people's lives and successes. Share experiences. Small talk is a good way to get acquainted. If a girl you'd like to get to know is wearing a sweater you like, for example, you could compliment her and ask where she bought it.

There are many different ways to make friends. At school, you'll probably find someone who shares your interests. Your friend may be somebody who lives on your street. You can also meet people and make friends if you join clubs where everyone has a common interest. You may find you have different friends who share different parts of your life.

What makes a friendship?

All kinds of things can bring two people together in a friendship. Often a friendship is based on some shared activity. If you're

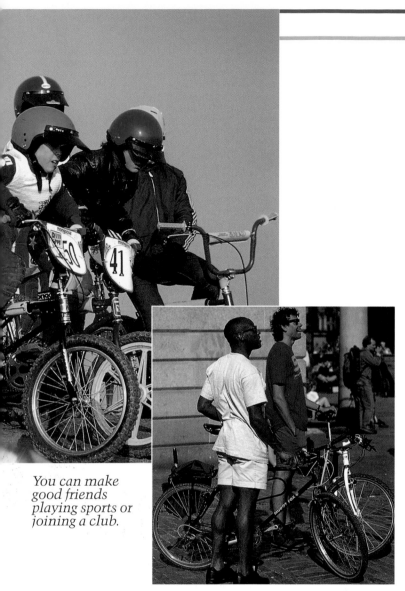

You can make good friends playing sports or joining a club.

have dozens of ideas that you want to discuss, but you may prefer not to raise some of them with parents or with the rest of your family. Yet you can always talk to your best friend. Best friends are going through the same experiences as you, and they understand how you feel.

Your best friend is likely to be somebody with whom you spend much of your free time. This friend will share good times and bad. This is the person you can laugh with, cry with, and share your secrets with. Teen-agers have many private concerns – relationships with parents, self-image, feelings about the opposite sex. A best friend can be counted on to explore these thoughts with you. A best friend is also someone you can trust.

Ups and downs

Friendship isn't always easy. Your best friend may drift away from you and become closer to someone else. If that happens, you'll probably be hurt and upset, and you may take a long time to get over it.

On the other hand, you may become interested in dating someone and not spend as much time with your best friend as you used to. Your friend may feel jealous and hurt.

But having a girlfriend or boyfriend doesn't mean that you have to desert your other friends. You should continue to see them. Talk to them about what is happening with you. A really good friend won't mind sharing your time with others.

Keep your friends

All your friends are precious, so working at friendship is worth the effort. A true friendship is a "give and take" relationship.

Friends must be able to trust each other. You can't expect friends to stick around forever if you keep letting them down. Even if you're busy with other things in your life, try to keep in touch with the friends you really value and let them know what you're doing. Listen to what's happening with them. Make sure they know that you care about them.

involved in a sport or hobby and enjoy the coaching, the competition, or the contact with other team or club members, it's easy to find a kindred spirit who shares your enthusiasm.

Sometimes you become friends when you feel a natural sympathy with someone else. You may be drawn to someone whose personality is similar to your own, someone who's shared some of the same experiences in life. Or your friend may be someone who acts more as a guide or teacher, encouraging you to try new ideas or venture into new experiences.

Best friends

A best friend is somebody you can talk to about anything and everything, someone with whom you have things in common and whose company you enjoy. At your age, you probably

Part of the group

Belonging to a group can make life a lot easier and a lot more fun. Everyone in the group may share a "private" language, a kind of code that only members of the group understand. You have "in" jokes, "in" clothes to wear, "in" places to visit or be seen at. It feels good to fit in and belong; it gives you an extra sense of security. The group makes you feel more self-confident because the members accept and like you. All the members of the group support each other.

Within a group of friends are usually recognizable roles. Some people are the leaders; others are the comics, the funny ones who crack all the jokes; still others are the fall guys, the ones who seem to be the butt of the jokes but can take it. And there are the easygoing members who just go along with what the others say. Does this sound like your group? Do any of these roles sound like yours?

Acting together

Of course, a close-knit group has to work out a way of making decisions so that everyone is happy about what the group is going to do. Often, all the members discuss things together and arrive at an answer together.

But sometimes the strongest members of the group make all the decisions. Although you joined the group because you generally like doing the same sorts of things as the others, you may sometimes find yourself being pressured into doing things that you don't want to do or that you feel are not right. This feeling is called peer pressure. Your peers are your equals – the friends in the group. At times you may feel they expect you to act in a certain way even though you don't really want to. People give into peer pressure for different reasons. They don't want to be ridiculed. They don't want to be thought of as "uncool." Most important, they don't want to be thrown out of the group.

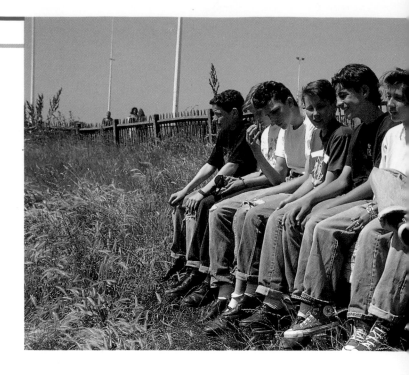

Taking things too far

Peer pressure is often harmless. But at other times, it is not. Some members of a group may think it's more important to conform to the rules of the group than to the laws of society. Many problems among teen-agers arise when members of a group urge each other to try drugs, smoke, drink alcohol, or commit acts of vandalism or even violence against other people. This kind of behavior, known as delinquent behavior, not only hurts the victims; it also hurts the individuals who carry it out and anyone associated with them.

Delinquency is most common in cities, where groups may become gangs. A new set of rules takes over on the "street." No one writes down these rules; they spring up as the group "needs" them. Often, poverty plays a strong part in the formation of gangs. But it is more complicated than that. People will do what they believe is best for themselves. For instance, if a young person feels it's better to drop out of school and earn money by selling drugs or running numbers, he or she may well drop out, especially if the group pressures him or her to do so. In the short term, this decision seems like smart thinking. But in the long term, it is not. Teens like this often end up addicted to drugs or in trouble with the police. At worst, they risk being murdered. Resisting peer pressure of this kind takes strength, but it's well worth the effort in the long run.

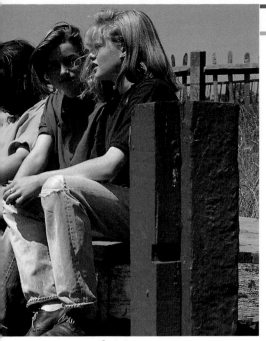

Many people get a lot of support from their group of friends.

If the members of a group get bored, they need to find something constructive to do.

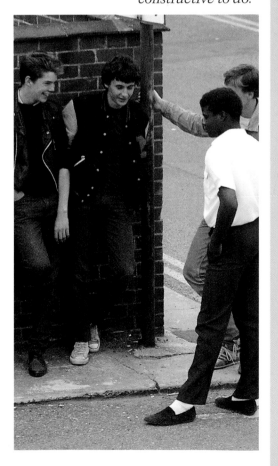

Gang violence

Young people growing up today are no strangers to violence. TV, movies, even major sports show violence as a matter of routine. In some schools, fights are daily events. In one study of high school students, 2 out of 10 had felt so fearful that they said they had carried a weapon to school for protection. Some schools have metal detectors to try to keep weapons out.

Much of this violence comes from gangs. In the United States, juvenile gangs involved in criminal activities are found mainly in low-income, declining neighborhoods of major cities. However, gangs are increasingly appearing in suburban areas and small towns. In many cases, the gang members share the same ethnic or racial identity.

Gang members may spend much of their time together loafing on street corners. But at other times, they engage in dangerous criminal activities, from stealing money and cars to drug abuse and drug dealing. Increasingly, such crime is accompanied by violence, especially involving guns. Conflict between rival gangs often leads to fighting and killing.

Young people join gangs for social and psychological as well as economic reasons. Little parental control, pessimism about their chances of succeeding in the mainstream of society, and lack of jobs all contribute to teen gang membership. Some teen-agers join gangs that tell them they protect their neighborhood. But that's not true. Very soon after joining a gang, new members will be asked to prove their loyalty by committing some act of violence against an innocent victim, often a person from the neighborhood. They also will be required to get involved in activities that raise money for the gang, most often by selling drugs and guns.

Resisting gangs is extremely difficult for many young people today. A teen-ager may try to keep out of their way. Or some teens may try to band together when they feel threatened. These are good survival techniques, but with the abundance of guns, they do not always work. In many cities, drive-by shootings hurt or kill innocent victims as well as rival gang members.

In one major city, however, grown men cruise the streets on Friday and Saturday nights for a different reason. They're volunteers looking for young people who are hanging out to give them a simple but important message: You don't have to join a gang. The men talk to the kids and determine what each young person is looking for. Is it friends? Excitement? Recreation? Then they take the teen-agers to a neighborhood gym, social club, or youth organization. In this way, the volunteers introduce the young people to places they can go to have fun and feel safe.

The opposite sex

As you may already have found out, the teen-age years are the time when boys begin to notice girls in a new way, and girls begin to notice boys in a new way. Opposites – in this case, the opposite sexes – attract.

Some people have many friends of the opposite sex, while others have few. There are many reasons you might find it hard or easy to form this kind of friendship.

Meeting

If, for example, you're the only girl in a family of brothers, you'll know a lot about boys. You'll understand how they think and know the things they like to do. You'll probably meet quite a few boys simply by being around when your brothers invite friends over. You therefore have a good chance to form friendships with boys.

On the other hand, you may have very little contact with the opposite sex. Perhaps you go to an all-girls or all-boys school. Perhaps you're an only child. Or your family may be very protective and strict about the freedom allowed to daughters, if not sons. Don't worry. There will be plenty of time to find out about the opposite sex and to form boy-girl friendships and relationships. Just be sure to let things happen naturally. Close

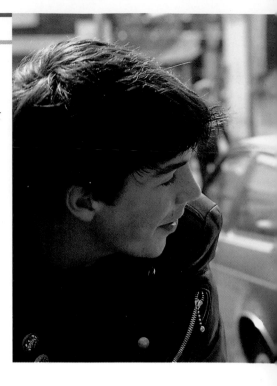

A friendship between a boy and a girl often arises from being involved in the same activities.

friendships usually arise from routine contact with friends at school, at parties, at sports events, or through introductions by families or friends.

What attracts you?

You may think that people are attracted only by each other's looks. That's not so. People are attracted to each other for many different reasons. You may like somebody who makes you laugh, who is easy to talk to, or who just makes you feel good to be you. Often people are attracted to those who have similar interests.

Another common misconception is that you have to be deeply in love with somebody of the opposite sex in order to have a special, close relationship with them. Many boys and girls are simply friends. Their relationship is more like brother and sister. To be happy and comfortable with somebody of the opposite sex, without feeling that you have to be in love with them, is a sign of maturity.

Don't be pressured!

Do all your friends have a girlfriend or boyfriend? If so, you may feel you should, too. But don't be pressured by your friends, and don't put pressure on yourself. Most important, you shouldn't feel inadequate because you

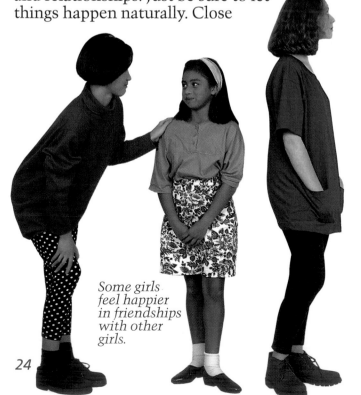

Some girls feel happier in friendships with other girls.

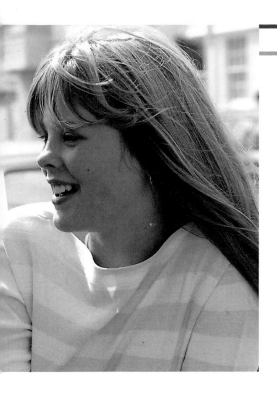

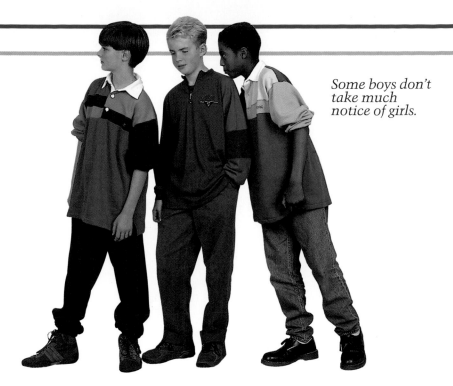

Some boys don't take much notice of girls.

don't have a girlfriend or boyfriend. Do what's best for you. You don't have to have a close relationship to be classified "normal"!
In fact, there's nothing wrong with not wanting to date at all. Perhaps you don't yet feel comfortable with people of the opposite sex and are happy having close friendships with people of your own sex. You may feel more confident going around in a crowd of friends. Either feeling is perfectly normal. Learning independence is an important part of growing up. If you are secure in yourself, you are far more likely to develop rewarding relationships than those who feel they can't exist without a partner.

Attracted to the same sex

It's not unusual for teen-agers to be attracted to people of the same sex, or even develop crushes on them. It is even fairly common for young boys – and, less frequently, for young girls – to stimulate each other sexually. Many teen-agers worry that this means they are homosexual. But such activity rarely indicates a homosexual preference. Usually, the young people are simply exploring their own emotional and sexual development.

Some teens, however, are truly homosexual. For a more in-depth discussion on homosexuality, read Volume 4 in this series, *Understanding Sexuality*.

Reader's experience

"At school, we all get along very well together. Sometimes we form pairs to do things. When I have a girl as my partner in that kind of situation, I'm fine. When I get out of school, though, it's a different story. I feel very nervous around girls. I just don't know what to say to them. I always think they're laughing at me.

"One of my friends started going out with a girl, and now he's fixed me up with her friend. He seems to find it easy to get along with girls. He told me to act like I do in class and I'll be fine. So I'm going to go out with them. I feel really nervous about it. I just wish we were in a classroom situation and not out on a date."
Joseph

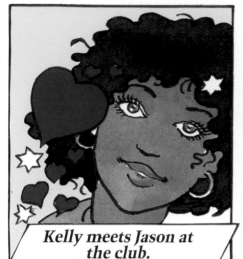

Kelly meets Jason at the club.

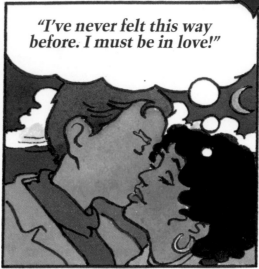

"I've never felt this way before. I must be in love!"

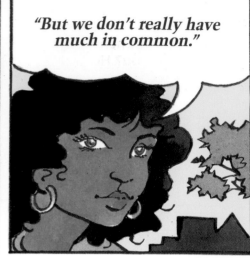

"But we don't really have much in common."

Falling in love

Some teens are in love with love. They have learned about love from television and movies, and they just can't wait to try it out for themselves. But love can take many different forms. One question a person must face is whether he or she is really in love at a particular time. For example, some people mistake physical desire for love. But love based only on physical attraction does not last long. A person may fall in love several times before developing a lasting, loving relationship with someone.

First encounters with love

One of your first experiences with love may be an infatuation. *Infatuation* comes from the Latin word *fatuus*, meaning "foolish." When you're infatuated, you allow your passion to overwhelm you — you are foolishly in love. You might adore somebody so much that you can't think about anything else. Your passion might even become an obsession.

A relationship based on infatuation is more about receiving than giving. Objects of infatuation are often unavailable, older people — a teacher, perhaps, or a movie star. People who are infatuated usually have an unrealistic view of their "idol." If they actually get a chance to meet and spend some time with the person, they can be disappointed that their idol is not as perfect as they imagined in their fantasies. However, an infatuation is a way of getting ready to handle a mature, two-way relationship.

To love somebody, you have to love and value yourself first. Once you can begin to understand your own feelings, you will be ready to start forming a close relationship with somebody else.

What does love feel like?

When you are falling in love, the whole world looks different. Everything glows. The weather is beautiful even if it is raining, and the most unpopular teacher at school suddenly seems bearable. You are filled with energy and happiness. That is the romantic side of love.

When you love someone, you are aware of that person's needs. When you make him or her happy, you are happy. As well as being physically attracted, the two of you are also best friends. You talk to each and have fun together. You enjoy being together as much as possible in many different situations and moods. You trust each other enough to reveal your emotions to each other. That is true love.

Breaking up

Sometimes feelings of love change. Perhaps, as time passes, the relationship is no longer as enjoyable. You can grow apart as you get older. Your interests and goals may lead you in separate directions. Although splitting up can be painful, be honest with each other. Clinging to a relationship that is not working out usually makes you feel worse in the long run than breaking it off.

HOW DO YOU GET OVER A BROKEN HEART?

What happens when your boyfriend or girlfriend falls "out of love" with you? He or she may want to be free – maybe even to see someone else. Such rejection hurts. You may feel that you did something wrong or you weren't good enough to be loved by that person. But consider the possibility that the decision may not have had a lot to do with you. People often break up because they're not ready for a serious relationship, even though they care about the other person. Still, being "rejected" may leave you feeling lonely, angry, and full of self-doubt. This is normal. And there are ways to get over it.

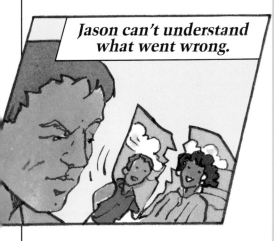

Jason can't understand what went wrong.

You can cry. You can voice your anger. You can talk to someone. You can stay busy. You can write down your feelings in a diary, a poem, or a song. You can believe your friends when they tell you how terrific you are.

Expressing your feelings is important. Just keep reminding yourself that you are lovable. After a while, you'll meet someone who is right for you.

Teen marriages

Some young people fall so deeply in love that they begin to consider marriage. The earliest age at which people may marry varies among countries and even among states in the United States.

In almost all states, both partners must be at least 18 years old to marry without their parents' permission. Most states allow people to marry as young as 16 with parental consent. A person under 16 may marry in some states if he or she has a judge's permission. However, people who are under 18 are generally not considered mature enough to take on the many responsibilities of marriage and parenthood.

People who marry before they are 18 years old are much more likely to have unsuccessful marriages than if they had waited until they were older. The divorce rate among American teens is one-and-a-half times the rate for people who marry after age 20. Why do so many teen marriages fail?

For a marriage to work, both partners must be emotionally and intellectually mature. Each also has to be willing to accept the other's faults. However, it usually takes time for two people in love to see each other realistically. Many teen-age marriages fail because the couples entered into them too quickly, before they had time to really get to know each other.

Teen-agers go through a lot of changes while they are developing their own identities. With all these changes, many teens find it hard to truly know who they themselves are. Think of how much harder it can be to know a partner!

Many 15- to 19-year-olds decide to marry not because they are in love, but to escape an unhappy home or because the girl is pregnant. Marriages entered into for these reasons generally do not last. Even if a teen couple marries for love, marriage brings major emotional and financial obligations. A baby brings even more. Friends and parties may soon drop out of the picture for the teen-age couple. Many teen-age marriages cannot withstand the pressures of all these responsibilities.

What about the teen marriages that do last? They survive for the same reasons that any successful marriage lasts. First, a marriage is more likely to succeed if the partners know each other well before they marry. A couple is more likely to know each other well if they have *grown* into love over a period of time, rather than *fallen* into love suddenly. It is also more likely to succeed if both partners have completed school.

Once married, a couple is more likely to stay married not only if they love each other but also have mutual respect. Sharing interests and goals, communicating with each other, and being determined to make the marriage work are important qualities that contribute to a successful marriage – no matter what age the couple is.

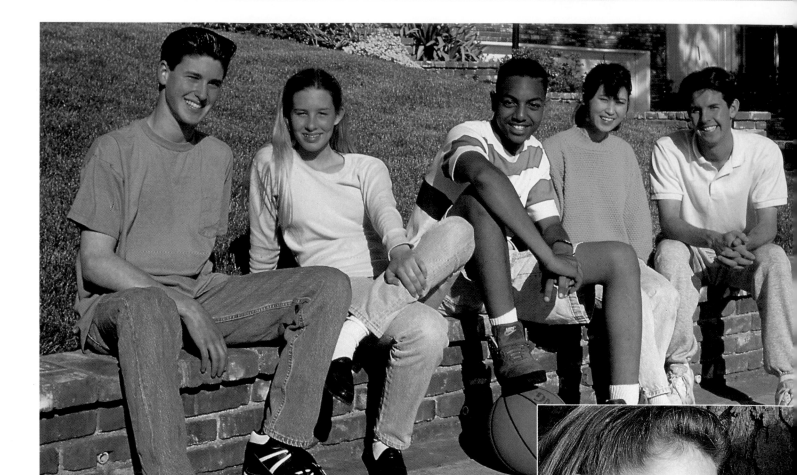

Many people prefer to meet friends of the other sex in a group.

Dating

Are you starting to think about dating? Or have you already been going out on dates? Many teens look forward to their first date.

What about your parents?

If your parents are like most parents, they'll probably have their own idea about when you're ready to date. Once you start dating, they also will probably want to meet the people you go out with and want you home by a certain time. You may want to do your own thing, but by following these guidelines, you'll show your parents that you really are mature enough to date.

If you like someone but your parents feel you're not old enough to date, ask them if you can invite your friend over to your home.

Group fun

Young people who start dating early often miss out on group activities. In fact, going out in a group is a good way to meet a particular boy or girl you may be interested in. When you go out in a group, you don't have to worry about the whole evening going wrong. There's always somebody to talk to. When you're together with friends, you probably won't feel so shy. And if you feel attracted to one of the members of the group, you'll be able to approach the person in a natural, more spontaneous way. Your first words may not be anything special – just a superficial greeting. But if the other person seems interested, you'll soon be having a more meaningful conversation.

A close relationship can grow out of a good friendship.

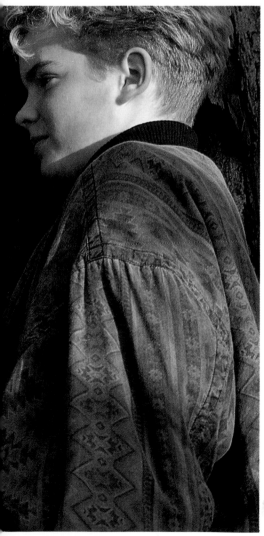

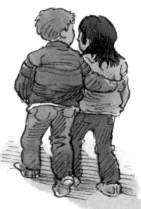

Making the first move

When you meet someone you like and think you'd like to date him or her, you may have to make the first move. When your parents were young, the boy usually did the asking, but today it's more acceptable for the girl to take the initiative. Some girls say their boyfriend was so shy that nothing would have happened if they hadn't asked him out.

The first time you ask someone out, you may be worried that he or she will turn you down. Don't let that stop you from asking. Be confident. Think of an interesting thing to do on your date – something you'll both enjoy. You may be tempted to ask someone out because they're really popular or good-looking even though you really don't have that much in common. But dating a good-looking, popular person doesn't guarantee that you'll have a good time.

Being turned down

If someone declines your invitation, don't get discouraged. The person may be interested in someone else or may already have a date for that night. He or she may happily accept your second invitation, so don't be afraid to try again.

Double-dating

A halfway stage between going out with a group and going out on a one-to-one basis is to double-date. When two couples go out together, you get some of the benefits of going out in groups, such as more people to contribute to the conversation. But you also get to enjoy being out with that "special someone."

When it doesn't work out

Feelings sometimes change quite rapidly. You may feel attracted to somebody and can't wait to go out with him or her, but when you do, the person may turn out to be different from what you expected. Going out with someone should be enjoyable. If things don't work out between you and a date, it simply means that you are not the right people for each other.

Sexual aggression

You may already have discovered many good things about being a teen-ager, such as becoming more independent. However, your new-found freedom may make you vulnerable to unwanted sexual attention, even sexual assault. It may surprise you to know that studies among adults in the United States report that anywhere from 14 to 33 per cent of women and 3 to 16 per cent of men have said that they experienced some kind of sexual assault when they were growing up. It's naive to believe that nothing bad can ever happen to you.

Sexual harassment

Sexual harassment can take different forms. Being touched or rubbed in a sexual way when you are moving along or standing in a crowded place is one kind of harassment. Yet this kind of behavior doesn't always involve strangers. When we are young, we are used to being hugged and caressed by our parents, by relatives, and by family friends. Sadly, some of these people may take advantage of a young person's trust and affection. They may love a young person, but still can't resist touching him or her in a sexual way. If you feel that your body is being touched and explored in an intimate way that you don't feel comfortable with, or if things are said to you that embarrass or upset you, make sure you tell someone you trust.

Sexual harassment can also take the form of flashing or obscene phone calls. Flashers are people, usually men, who expose their genitals in public. If a flasher exposes himself to you, move away quickly, join other people who are nearby, or try to attract attention by shouting. Obscene phone calls can also be upsetting, especially if you're alone at home when you receive one. The best tactic is to hang up at the first obscene word. If the calls continue, report them to the police or to the phone company.

Being on the receiving end of sexual harassment is not your fault. It is the result of someone else's problem with his or her sexuality. If you are sexually harassed, don't be afraid to tell someone about it. The person needs to stop this behavior, and you need to be left alone.

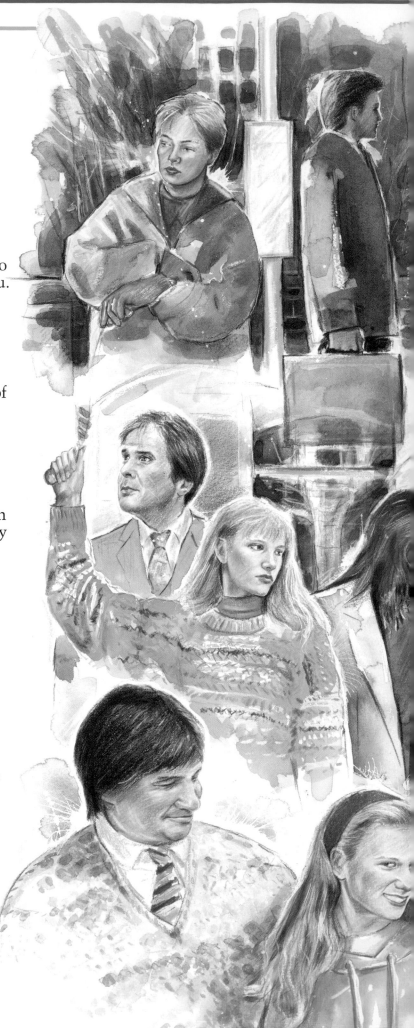

Rape

Rape is forcing someone to have sexual intercourse. A rapist is usually a man, and a rape victim is usually a woman or girl. However, men and boys can be rape victims. In fact, rape is considered a crime of violence, not of sex.

You may think a rapist is a stranger who leaps out of bushes and attacks someone. This is sometimes the case. However, according to one survey, about half of all rapes occur between people who know each other. This is called acquaintance rape.

To reduce the risk of an attack from an unknown person, don't walk alone at night or in dangerous areas. Make sure you lock all the doors when you are home alone, and don't let strangers into your home at any time.

You may want to carry an alarm that makes a high-pitched shrieking noise. If you are attacked, you can use it to scare off the attacker. Or you may be able to scream or shout to attract help. You may be able to poke your attacker's eyes. However, if your attacker is in control, or threatening you with a weapon, it is sometimes best to try to talk. Concentrate on getting a description of the person to give to the police once you are free.

Acquaintance rape can take place in a car or at a party—even in your own home. If someone asks you to have sex, make sure your answer is clear. If you say no, and are forced into sex against your will, the act is rape. It's possible to be raped and not even know it. Someone can slip a drug into your drink, causing you to do something you wouldn't ordinarily do and not remember it later. While some of these drugs turn blue in liquid, others are colorless. If you feel at risk, don't accept any opened drink, especially from strangers.

If you are raped, report it to the police as soon as possible. You should also get medical attention immediately. You may also feel the need to talk to a trusted friend or family member.

Telling your story

Don't be afraid to tell a sympathetic adult about a sexual assault as soon as it happens. You may worry that people won't believe you or that they will blame you for what happened, but if you don't report it, the experience could haunt and disturb you for many years.

A rape victim will be physically and emotionally upset. A doctor can treat a rape victim and keep him or her under observation until any physical wounds are completely healed. The psychological damage may take longer to heal, though. It may be very hard for a female rape victim to trust a man again. The more a rape victim can talk about the experience with people who can help, the sooner the emotional wounds can heal.

Rape is also extremely traumatic for boys and young men. They must deal not only with the physical and emotional trauma of the actual assault, but also with the fact that their attacker was another male. They may have feelings of guilt or weakness because they weren't able to successfully defend themselves. If they can accept the fact that *anyone* can be a victim of rape, they will probably find it easier to heal.

Smoking

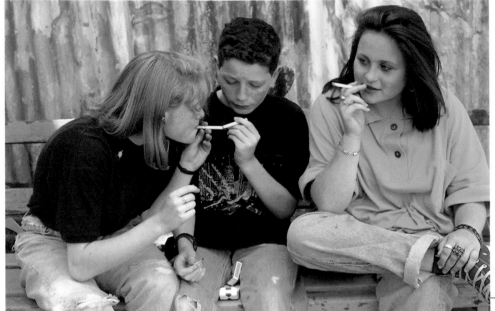

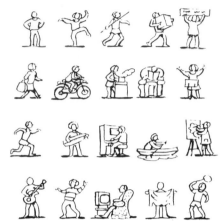

It's easy to think of many habits that are more worthwhile than smoking.

So you've decided not to smoke. That's great! You'll live longer, breathe easier, feel better, and save yourself thousands of dollars.

Some young people think that smoking will make them look grown-up and cool. They may also think it's a way of joining the crowd. These young people smoke because their friends pressure them to do so. Some teens may be copying parents who smoke, or other adults whom they respect. At one time, this imitation would have been accepted as normal. But in the last 30 years, attitudes about smoking have changed. Smoking is now banned in many public places so that other people don't have to breathe in smokers' choking tobacco smoke. This passive smoking can damage a person's health just as smoking can.

Smoking is one of the hardest habits to break. Cigarette smoke contains nicotine, a highly addictive drug, in addition to thousands of other chemicals, many of which have been linked to the development of disease. One of every five deaths in the United States is due to smoking.

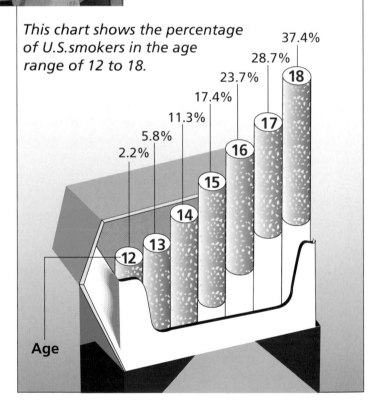

This chart shows the percentage of U.S. smokers in the age range of 12 to 18.

2.2%
5.8%
11.3%
17.4%
23.7%
28.7%
37.4%

12
13
14
15
16
17
18

Age

Quitting

If you already smoke, decide to stop smoking and stop today – even if you're halfway through a pack. Of course, quitting will be difficult, but your doctor can help you quit smoking and stay smoke free. Don't talk about tomorrow or the future. You are in control of your own life and can do what you want today.

Smoking-related illnesses

There's no doubt that smoking damages your health. The toxic substances in cigarette smoke include nicotine, carbon monoxide, and tar. Nicotine is the substance in tobacco that causes addiction. It is a stimulant that brings on an increase in pulse rate and blood pressure. Carbon monoxide is a poisonous gas. Other substances in cigarette smoke irritate the delicate linings of the air passages.

The air passages in your body are lined with mucus, which traps foreign particles. Small hairs called cilia then push the mucus back up the air passages. You get rid of the mucus by blowing your nose or coughing and spitting. However, when cigarette smoke is inhaled, the cilia stop working and no longer prevent the tar and nicotine in the smoke from getting into the lungs. The cilia eventually stop working altogether, making it easy for infection to set in and harder for the body to clear the mucus and infection out.

Chronic bronchitis can occur when the irritants in cigarette smoke are inhaled over a long period of time. The sufferer has a bad, phlegmy cough, especially in the mornings, and may get breathless easily.

Smoking is the principal cause of emphysema, an illness in which the smaller airways become blocked. The walls of the lungs' air sacs are gradually destroyed, so the lungs cannot efficiently take in oxygen or remove carbon dioxide. The victim feels tight in the chest and always short of breath.

Cigarette smoke can cause certain cells in the lungs to turn into cancer cells. These multiply, destroying healthy lung tissue and sometimes spreading through the body to start new cancerous growths. Lung cancer is not easy to treat because it is often not diagnosed in its early stages.

Apart from lung cancer, smokers can also suffer from cancer of the mouth, esophagus, larynx, bladder, and pancreas. Smoking is also a factor in the development of cervical cancer in women.

Nicotine increases blood pressure and pulse rate. Other substances in cigarette smoke speed up the development of blockages that can lead to a heart attack. Smokers are twice as likely to have heart disease as nonsmokers.

Smokeless tobacco, which is chewed rather than smoked, can cause tooth and gum damage, as well as cancer of the mouth, including the tongue, cheek, and gum.

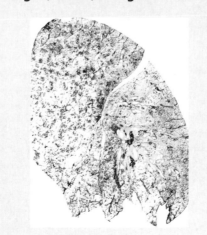

A lung damaged by smoking looks like this. A normal lung is pink.

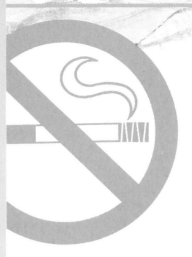

SAY NO TO TOBACCO

Smoke stinks. Far from making you seem mature, the smell of smoke on your breath and clothes will turn many people off.

Someone who smokes 20 cigarettes a day – one pack – loses about 5.5 minutes of life expectancy for each cigarette smoked.

Nicotine is a poisonous and addictive drug.

The chances of dying of cancer of the lung or larynx, emphysema, or heart disease increase when you smoke.

Smokers "burn" a great deal of money. In many countries, cigarettes are heavily taxed.

A smoker's skin wrinkles earlier and deeper than that of a nonsmoker. Smokers also have more wrinkles than nonsmokers.

Pregnant women who smoke run a higher risk of miscarriage and have babies with lower birth weights.

Alcohol

Many adults enjoy drinking alcohol in moderation.

But many teen-agers are pressured to drink with their friends at parties. After all, images of people in their 20's drinking beer and having fun abound on TV commercials. It's easy to associate drinking with grown-up fun. But teen-agers are legally underaged where alcohol is concerned. Alcoholic beverages cannot legally be sold to people under the age of 21 in any state of the United States.

Alcohol is a drug

Even adults who can and do drink in moderation must realize that alcohol is a drug. In fact, it is the most widely used drug among both adults and teen-agers. It is also the most frequently abused drug among both adults and teen-agers. Alcohol affects many of the body's organs. In some people, drinking can lead to alcohol addiction, known as alcoholism.

If you choose to use alcohol, you need to be aware of its effects and the potential dangers involved.

Never drink and drive

Approximately 40 percent of all automobile-related deaths are caused by drunk drivers. For years people have been told not to drink and drive. And yet some people still do. The alcohol in the body of a drunk driver clouds judgment and reduces his or her reaction time. In addition, people who are drunk are less likely to wear their seat belts. If they have an accident, the alcohol in their body will make medical treatment of any injury more difficult. But most important, a drunk driver is a real danger to other drivers and pedestrians—a potential killer. Remember, there is no way you can drink and drive safely.

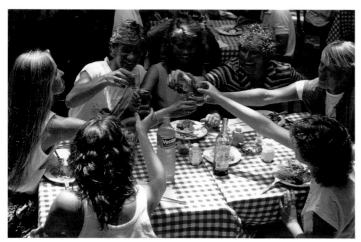

Drinking is often shown as being fun.

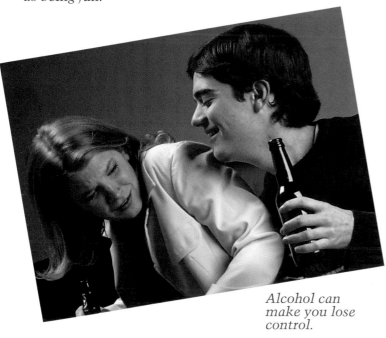

Alcohol can make you lose control.

Nearly half the car-related deaths in the U.S. are caused by drunk drivers.

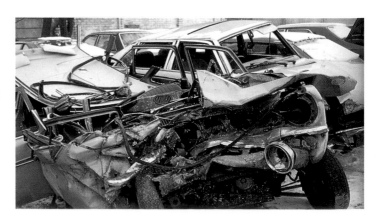

ALCOHOL AND ITS EFFECTS

Alcohol is, in fact, a mild poison. It begins to be absorbed into the bloodstream as soon as it reaches the stomach. Absorption is slower if food is in the stomach. Once inside the bloodstream, alcohol passes to the liver, where it is removed from the blood and broken down. But the liver can process only a certain, limited amount of pure alcohol each hour. Nearly all the remaining alcohol a person has drunk continues to circulate in the bloodstream until the liver can break it down. The amount the liver can process depends on many individual factors: a person's size, weight, gender, genetic history, and so on. On average, the liver of a 150-pound

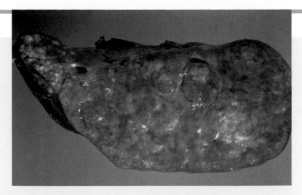

Heavy drinking causes cirrhosis of the liver.

(68-kilogram) man can process only about 7 grams of pure alcohol each hour. This is a relatively small amount – about half a glass of beer.

When alcohol reaches your brain, you may immediately feel more relaxed or even light-headed. You may feel like taking risks because alcohol lowers your inhibitions and clouds your judgment. It also makes some people feel aggressive. Your

actions become clumsy, and your speech may become slurred. If you continue to drink, you might experience double vision or even lose consciousness.

Later, you may suffer from a hangover, which is a mild form of withdrawal from alcohol. With a hangover, you have a headache and feel tired and nauseated. A hangover reminds you that drinking too much is bad for your body.

Is drinking really necessary?

Of course, you want to act grown-up when you're out with your friends. But you don't have to drink alcohol to do so. Many people – including many adults – simply don't like the taste of alcohol. Others don't like the effect even one glass has on them. Don't let friends pressure you to drink if you don't want to. Deciding what's best for you and sticking to your decision is the most grown-up act of all.

When drinking becomes a problem

Prolonged drinking can damage a person physically, mentally, and socially. One survey reported that in 1991 about 4 per cent of high school seniors in the United States had had at least one drink every day in the month before the survey; many more had drunk heavily at least once in that time. If you have a friend whose drinking worries you, try to get help for the person. Talking to your parents or a school counselor might be a start. Or, if a member of your own family is an alcoholic, you yourself could use help. Such groups as Alcoholics Anonymous for alcoholics, Al-Anon for families and friends of alcoholics, and Alateen for teen-age daughters and sons of alcoholics can help.

Beer is about 3 to 6 per cent alcohol, wine about 10 to 20 per cent, and "hard" liquor about 40 to 50 per cent. However, 12 oz. (355 ml) of beer, 5 oz. (148 ml) of wine, and 1.5 oz. (44 ml) of 80-proof liquor have about the same amount of alcohol.

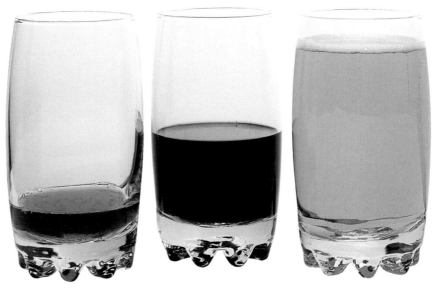

Drug abuse

All medicines are drugs. Your doctor may prescribe drugs if you have an infection or a condition such as asthma. But not all drugs are medicines. Alcohol is a drug, and nicotine is a drug. These are drugs that do you no good at all. Using an illegal drug or misusing a medicinal drug is drug abuse.

Many young people who experiment with drugs do so out of curiosity, for a thrill, to rebel, or because their friends use drugs. In fact, young people are usually introduced to drugs by their friends. When a friend offers you a chance to have some "fun" with drugs and points out that everyone is doing it, it's natural to wonder what the experience is like. Your friend may tell you stories about how wonderful the drugs will make you feel. What he or she won't tell you is how addictive the drugs are, how many thousands of teen-agers do lasting damage to their bodies by using drugs, and how many people die from continued drug abuse.

Side effects

In addition to the damage drugs can cause to your body, all drug abusers are in danger of suffering from side effects. Drug abusers need professional guidance and medical treatment.

Certain drugs can bring on confusion, drowsiness, and frightening hallucinations. A person on drugs puts himself or herself in danger of having an accident. Many drugs dull the reflexes, making it impossible to drive a car safely. Cocaine, even in small amounts, can cause sudden death in some young people because it produces an irregular heartbeat. Some drugs can interfere with breathing, and if someone accidentally overdoses, he or she may become unconscious or even die. Several drugs cause a loss of appetite, which can lead to other health problems. Of course, a child born to a woman who takes drugs can have serious physical and psychological problems.

Be strong

Drug abuse is not only physically harmful, it's illegal. Simple possession of certain amounts, in addition to selling drugs, can get a teen-ager in serious trouble with the law. Work out ahead of time how you will react if someone offers you a drug. Don't be pressured into changing your mind.

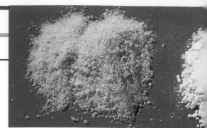
amphetamines

Amphetamines (speed, uppers, meth, crystal)

Yellowish crystal or powder but commonly obtained in pill or capsule form. Some amphetamines are prescribed for medical disorders. Can be sniffed or injected. Makes people hyperactive, alert, and irritable, but depression and difficulty with sleep can follow. Heavy use can produce feelings of persecution.

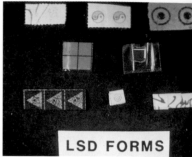
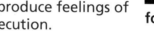
forms of LSD

MDMA (Ecstasy, E)

An amphetamine that can cause hallucinations similar to LSD in addition to amphetamine effects.

heroin

Cannabis (marijuana, pot, dope, hash, grass)

Hard, resinous material or leafy herbal mixture. Smoked in a joint or pipe. Distinctive herbal smell. Some effects are like those of alcohol.

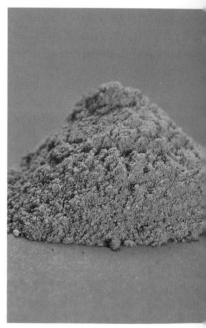

Cocaine (coke, blow, snow)

A white powder, commonly sniffed. Can be injected or smoked. Similar effects to amphetamines but more likely to lead to dependence. Crack cocaine is an especially dangerous, highly addictive form.

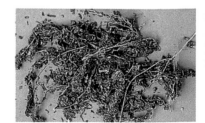
herbal cannabis

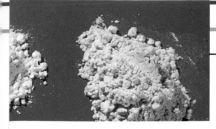

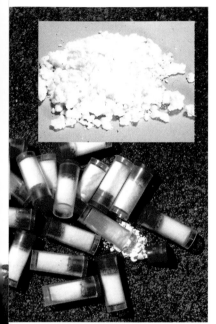

cocaine and crack cocaine

ecstasy

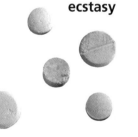

Different drugs are available in different parts of the world. They do not always look the same.

Heroin (smack, scag, H, horse)

Off-white or brown powder. Can be sniffed, injected, or smoked. Produces initial euphoria followed by drowsiness. Overdose can cause unconsciousness and death. Frequent use results in addiction.

LSD (acid)

Tablets and small paper or gelatin squares. Taken by mouth. Effects are unpredictable and range from excitement to panic and fear. Hallucinations. Recurrent "flashbacks" may also occur.

Mescaline (peyote)

Hallucinogenic drug obtained from certain forms of cactus. Usually smoked or eaten.

"Date-Rape" drugs (GHB, Rohypnol)

Cause sedation and memory loss. Might be slipped into someone's drink without his or her knowledge.

Psilocybin (magic mushroom)

Type of mushroom containing a substance like LSD. Produces hilarity, overexcitement, and, with high doses, dreamlike images.

Barbiturates (downers, reds)

Prescribed for epilepsy, but when abused have a similar effect to alcohol and increased effect when taken with alcohol. Withdrawal may result in seizures.

Inhalants

Inhalant sniffing ("huffing") describes breathing in chemicals found in household cleaning products as well as in aerosols, glues, thinners, and gases. Inhalants are addictive. Accidental overdoses are common and can result in death.

Oral narcotics (morphine, oxycodone, hydrocodone, etc.)

Prescribed for patients with severe acute and chronic pain. When abused, they have similar effects to heroin and are highly addictive.

Benzodiazepines (Valium, Xanax, Ativan, etc.)

Prescribed for patients with anxiety disorders. When abused, they have similar effects to alcohol and can be fatal if taken with alcohol. These drugs are highly addictive. Withdrawal may take several weeks and may cause seizures.

Drug users risk catching diseases, including HIV and hepatitus, if they share syringes.

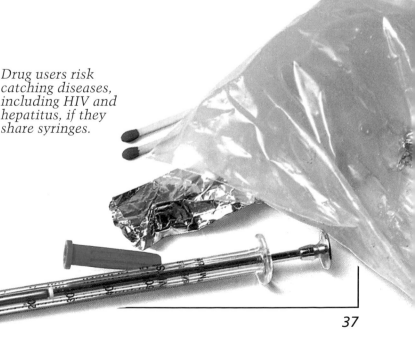

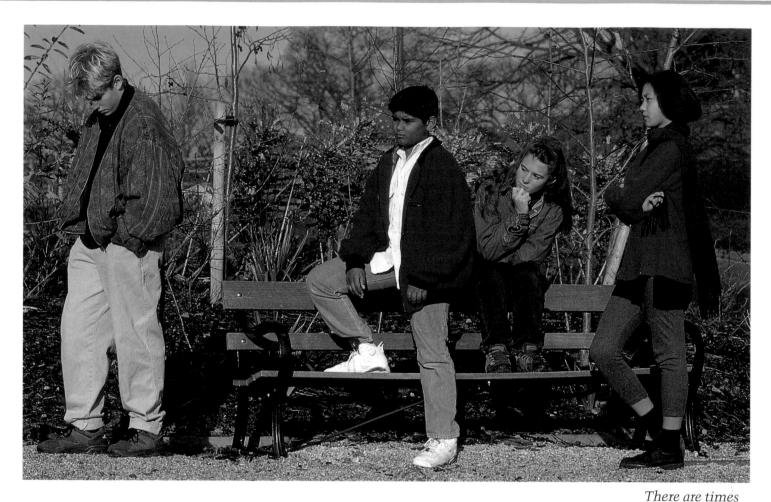

There are times when you have to control your temper.

Anger and frustration

Do you feel angry sometimes? Of course you do. Everyone does. Why? Because you are afraid of something? Perhaps you are worried about an exam or your grade-point average. Fear can often be disguised as anger. Or perhaps someone you know is ill. You are angry because it's unfair. You may feel frustrated because you think no one understands you or because you can't get what you need. As with fear, frustration often turns into anger.

When you feel frustrated or angry, your body produces a hormone called adrenalin that helps you deal with the situation. But if your body frequently reacts this way – in other words, if you are often angry or frustrated – you may be putting yourself under stress.

Dealing with anger

Anger is natural, but you must express it in a mature way. One good way to handle anger is to pinpoint its cause. Talk to your family or friends about it. That way, you'll relieve the pressure of built-up anger. Discussing what's bothering you is often the best way of finding a solution to it. Your family or friends may see what you need to do – and help you do it.

Bottling up your anger is never healthy. You need to vent your anger, but screaming, throwing things, pouting, or giving others the silent treatment is not the best way to do it. You'll find that vigorous exercise is good for letting off steam. Sometimes crying can make you feel better. Try going for a long walk by yourself. Or go to a place where you won't disturb anyone and have a good shout!

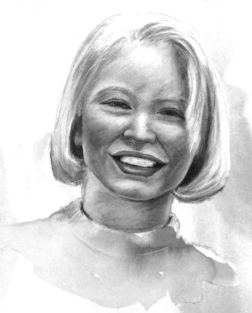

"There's a boy at school who has everything. He lives in an enormous house and has his own personal minibike and a whole room of computer games. He's so rich that he can just go out and buy anything he wants. My brother says I shouldn't envy him because being rich doesn't always make you happy. I don't know if I believe him, though. I wouldn't mind being rich!"
Adri

"When my friend is mad at me, I try not to care. There's no point in answering back. If I do, an argument soon starts, and that makes things worse. I try to walk away, or talk about something else."
Alice

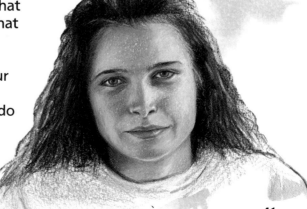

"My brother used to have a terrible temper. I was scared of him sometimes. He stormed around the house, slamming doors and shouting at us for no reason at all. Then he would go out for a long run and come back feeling better. But when he got on the cross-country team, he began to change. He seemed to find it easier to control his temper. Now he's the coolest brother on our street!"
Gloria

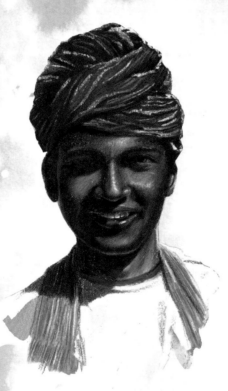

"I have a younger sister who's 5. I don't like her at all. She's really spoiled and gets everything she wants. Because she looks pretty and sweet, she gets all the attention, and I'm left out. My parents always say they love us equally, but it's hard to believe sometimes. I just wish my sister would grow up quickly."
Ciara

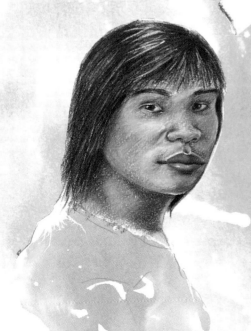

"My dad gets furious when he sees the amount of garbage that people throw away. He says that at least half of it could be recycled. Last year he helped start a recycling program in our town. He said that instead of complaining, it was better to do something positive with his anger and frustration. He's certainly done that."
D'Andre

Mood swings

Do you sometimes feel happy one minute and sad the next? These sudden changes of mood are a normal part of growing up. One cause of mood swings is your hormones, which are also responsible for the physical changes you're going through.

You're changing from a child into a young adult, and new experiences are changing your view of the world. You may be excited and stimulated by what you discover. But you might also feel torn because you no longer enjoy the same things that you used to. Although you really want to grow up, you may feel sad about leaving behind some aspects of your childhood. After all, wasn't it great when others took responsibility for your life, when your parents were perfect, when a new toy could make your day? Life is more complicated now.

Some teens find it easy to blame the people around them for their state of mind. Perhaps you're feeling frustrated with your parents because they don't seem to understand you anymore. Maybe you don't enjoy spending time with your family the way you used to. You may feel differently about your childhood friends too. Some may now seem juvenile and annoying. But blaming others for your moods does not help.

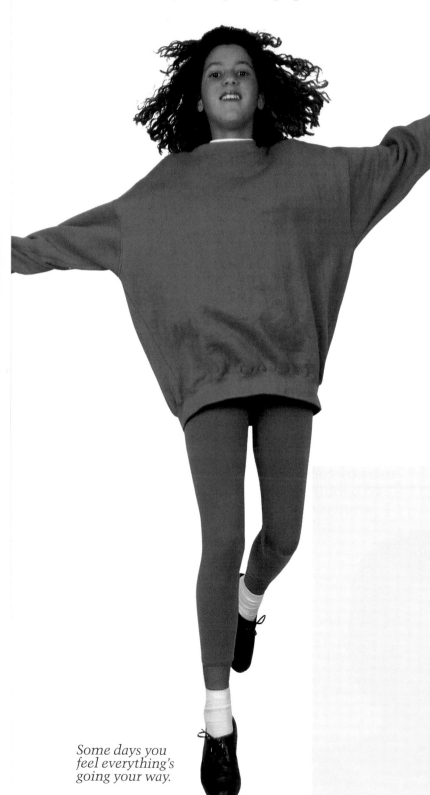

Some days you feel everything's going your way.

GOOD MOODS
Sometimes you may feel totally happy for no particular reason. Everything in the world is going your way. You're feeling good about yourself and your ability to deal with life, with people, and with change. What a great feeling! When you're in a mood like this, make the most of it. Enjoy every second of it!

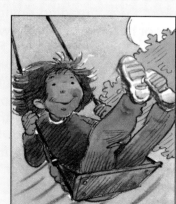

Coping with your moods

Although you can't avoid bad moods altogether, you can control your reaction to them. Don't blame others, but don't blame yourself either. When you suddenly find yourself in a bad mood, try to think back over time until you hit on the moment when things first began to feel wrong. The reason behind your mood swing may surprise you.

For example, one afternoon somebody may take your seat on the school bus. You become angry and upset, even though it's nothing serious. Your friends think you're silly for getting upset, and when you think about it afterward, you agree. You probably also admit to yourself that losing your seat wasn't the real problem at all. Perhaps it simply triggered other thoughts. You began to think it showed that people take you for granted. These feelings are at the core of your reaction.

Take positive action

Finding the reason behind your bad moods should help you cope with them. You can take action to make yourself feel better.

If you feel moody, go for a walk and take a little time to be by yourself. When you've thought things over, you may be ready to talk to somebody. Some people find physical activity helps a bad mood. Try tidying your room or playing with the dog. Doing something simple and undemanding for a while may make all the difference.

If certain people or situations put you in a bad mood, try to avoid them. It's worth telling people that you're in a bad mood and would rather be left alone. People who try to make you have a good time when you don't feel like it may make your mood worse. Or you may end up putting them in a bad mood!

Observing other people's moods may help you understand your own. For example, you might be out with your best friend, who is usually good fun. Today, however, your friend is moody and quiet. You're both having a lousy time. It's probably a good idea to go your separate ways and get in touch with each other later to talk about what's wrong. Let your friend know you've felt the same way at times.

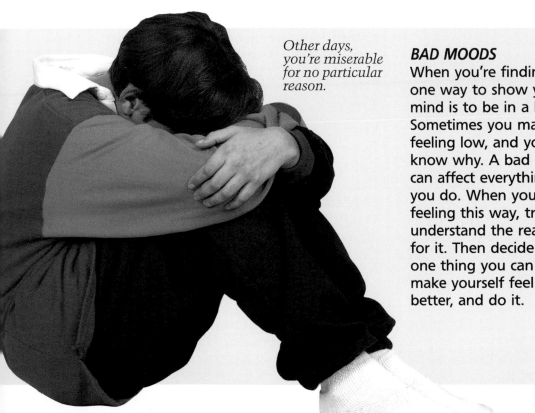

Other days, you're miserable for no particular reason.

BAD MOODS
When you're finding life difficult, one way to show your state of mind is to be in a bad mood. Sometimes you may wake up feeling low, and you don't even know why. A bad mood can affect everything you do. When you're feeling this way, try to understand the reason for it. Then decide on one thing you can do to make yourself feel better, and do it.

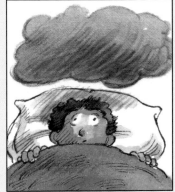

Emotional problems

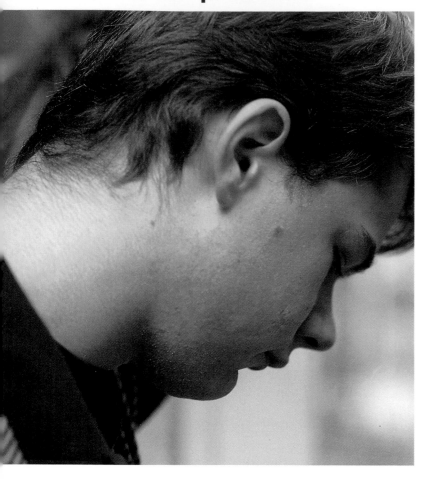

Depression can make you feel isolated.

Any depression that lasts longer than a few weeks should be taken seriously. Don't be discouraged from seeking treatment by someone who says, "You'll get over it; it's not really a problem." That's bad advice. Depression may stem from a medical problem. If so, your doctor can treat it, probably with medication. If your depression turns out to have an emotional rather than physical cause, your doctor may recommend exercise, meditation, or activities such as volunteer work. Perhaps therapy might be a good idea. Some neighborhoods offer support groups for teen-agers. If your doctor doesn't know of any, a school counselor or member of the clergy may.

Suicide

Perhaps you have a good friend who is very depressed. Maybe this friend has mentioned fantasies about suicide. Always take threats of suicide seriously. Your friend needs help. If he or she can talk things over with friends, it's a good start. But people who are seriously depressed need professional help. Urge your friend to see a doctor. Anyone who talks about committing suicide needs medical attention immediately. If your friend refuses, tell an adult you trust about the situation.

Stress

Stress is not always bad for the human body. In fact, we need some stress to keep us stimulated. But when someone is under stress for a long time, they may suffer. Problems pile up, and they feel powerless to deal with them.

When you're under stress, your body produces the hormone adrenalin. Adrenalin makes your heart beat faster and your breathing rate increase. These physical reactions aren't harmful in themselves. But if high-level stress lasts for a while, your body can suffer a stress overload. The result may be serious physical effects such as headaches and stomach ulcers, high blood pressure or heart attacks.

Depression

Losing interest in life can be an indication of depression. When you are depressed, you may feel there's no reason to get through today or to be excited about tomorrow. You may have problems sleeping or feel tired all the time. You may lose your appetite or overeat. Everything may seem hopeless and bleak. Your family and friends may tell you to "just cheer up." It's not that simple, however. You may feel frustrated and angry with yourself for not being able to snap out of it.

Rage, self-hate, and anxiety, if kept inside, can make you very depressed. Depression is not just an adult problem. Nowadays, more and more teen-agers are suffering from real depression, often aggravated by the problems of drugs, alcohol, pressure at school, or the breakup of the family. There are physical reasons for depression as well. Sometimes a chemical imbalance in the body can cause it.

If you think you are under stress, do two things right away. One, talk to somebody about your problems. Two, allow yourself some time each day to relax. You need to feel that you are in charge of your life, not that your life is in charge of you. You may need to accept that there are some things you're just not able to do. Decide what's most important to you.

POSSIBLE SIGNS OF DEPRESSION

You often feel tired.
You have trouble falling asleep.
You wake up in the middle of the night and cannot get back to sleep.
Routine actions seem exhausting.
It's hard to get up in the morning.
You lose your appetite.
Your appetite increases.
You are accident-prone.
You find it hard to make decisions.
You cry a lot without knowing why.
You feel hopeless.

POSSIBLE SIGNS OF STRESS

You are bad-tempered and snap at people.
You have frequent headaches.
You have stomach pains and nausea, or constant "butterflies" in your stomach.
You find it hard to get to sleep.
You wake early.
You find it hard to concentrate at school.
You cry a lot.
You lose your appetite.
Your appetite increases.
You bite your nails.

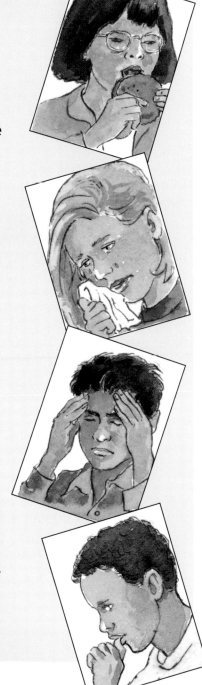

Dealing with stress

Not everyone deals with stress equally well. People who are confident about coping with life's problems manage better than people who feel helpless. If you can persuade yourself that you can deal with problems, you'll manage stress better.

Supportive family and friends can help you in times of stress. That works in reverse as well. If one of your family members or friends is under stress, support the person. Show him or her that you care.

Setting goals

Some people regain a sense of control over their lives by setting and meeting goals. A goal doesn't have to be grandiose. If you decide you want to be fluent in Portuguese by next month, for example, you're setting yourself up for failure. Think of something that would make your life easier. Are you always rushed in the morning? Set a goal of getting up as soon as the alarm rings. Do you have no time for yourself? Set a goal of getting a half hour of quiet time each night. Setting and achieving realistic goals can help you feel good about yourself.

Some good advice for beating the blues

Get regular exercise. Physical exercise is good for the mind as well as for the body. It gives you more energy, and it is a good way to work out anger. Studies have shown that if you exercise regularly, your body creates higher levels of beta endorphins, natural hormones that help you feel better about yourself. If you are physically tired, you may find it easier to fall asleep.

Don't hold things in. Have a good cry if you can. Talk to someone who will listen.

It may seem difficult to do when you're down, but make a list of all the things you really enjoy in life. At first, you may think you have nothing to write. Persevere and you'll probably surprise yourself. Give yourself something to look forward to every day – little things, such as talking with a good friend, watching a favorite video, walking through a park, or reading a magazine.

47

Exam pressure

When you're a teen-ager, tests occupy a very important part in your life. Some tests are midterm or final exams that affect your grades at school. Other types are college entrance examinations that will decide whether you go to college and, if so, what college you attend.

Some cultures emphasize education more than others do, and parents vary in what they expect from their children. You may feel a great deal of pressure for you to succeed, both at school and at home. You may find that you spend a lot of time worrying about school and exams. Of course, if you work hard at school and succeed, your family will be pleased with you, and you'll be pleased with yourself. Yet too much pressure to succeed at school may lead to stress-related illness.

Whether you excel at schoolwork or get average grades, you *will* feel pressure to stay in high school until you get a diploma – and with good reason. Your education will benefit you greatly when you go to get a job. This is particularly true today, when fewer and fewer positions are available to unskilled workers. In general, workers with high-school diplomas earn significantly more throughout their lives than those who drop out of high school, and workers with college educations earn significantly more than those with only a high-school diploma.

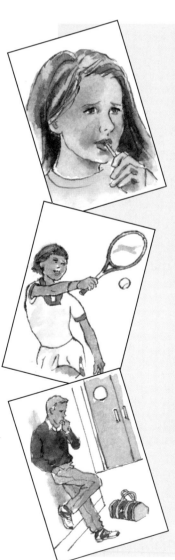

HOW TO SURVIVE EXAM PRESSURE

Try to study a little every day. Complete assignments as you receive them. Steady studying is more valuable than last-minute cramming. You're more likely to absorb facts and retain them if you study in this way.

Some books discuss special exam techniques. Why not check a few of these books out of the library to see if these techniques can help? Your teachers can also help and guide you. Some schools offer special classes on study skills.

Have you ever dreamed this dreadful nightmare: You walk into an examination room, turn over the paper, and your mind goes completely blank? This doesn't have to happen to you. Sometimes a teacher will show you exam papers from previous years so that you'll become familiar with the format and kinds of questions asked.

Can you spend the afternoon before a big exam playing basketball, swimming, or doing some other form of exercise? This might sound like a waste of time. But if you've studied all along, exercise may be better for you than a last-minute review. You'll sleep well and arrive at the exam feeling rested and relaxed.

Try not to turn up for an exam too early. Waiting around may make you more nervous.

Don't even think of cheating as an option. Cheating will make you think less of yourself. Self-esteem is closely linked to success, so cheating is self-defeating in the long run.

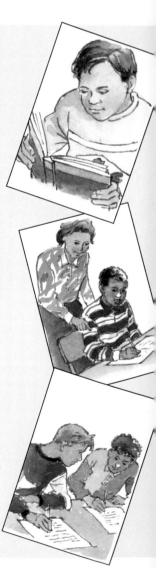

Steady study is better than last-minute cramming.

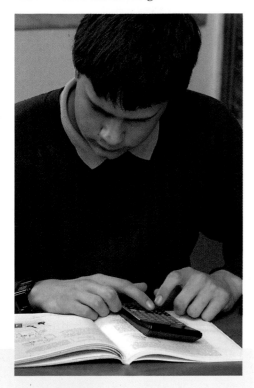

EXAM NERVES

Getting nervous before an exam is normal, even if you know you've studied hard. This nervousness shows itself in physical symptoms such as:

- restlessness
- talkativeness
- headaches
- stomachaches
- nausea
- sweaty hands
- racing heartbeat
- shaking hands
- dry mouth
- compulsive swallowing

If you experience any of these symptoms before an exam, you're not alone. However, they usually disappear once you've sat down and begun the exam. Try some deep breathing to calm your nerves. And remember, the other students are feeling the same way as you.

Examination pressures in two countries

High-school students in the United States must generally take one of two college entrance exams if they plan to enter college – the Scholastic Aptitude Test (SAT) or the American College Testing Program test (ACT). These tests can cause a great deal of tension, and some students buy special books or go to tutors to prepare for them.

However, in Japan placement-exam pressure begins even earlier. *Juken jigoku,* or examination hell, exists in Japan because nearly all 14-year-old students in junior high school wish to continue their education beyond 15, the age at which students may legally leave school. But Japan does not have enough low-cost, state-maintained senior high schools, so competition is stiff among 14-year-olds to get into the best upper school in their area. Indeed, most children experience "double schooling." Outside regular school hours, most Japanese students attend *juku,* or cram school, for about five hours a week in order to maximize their chances. However, once Japanese students have entered senior high school, they get only a short breathing space before *juken jigoku* starts again, as they prepare for entrance examinations to a university.

A recent survey showed that many young Japanese people love their studies. One girl wrote, "I will never forget the final words of a teacher when he retired from my high school last year: 'Life, until death, is study.'" Another wrote, "I don't think there are many students in countries other than Japan who are pushed into high school entrance exams, so I think that passing the exams is the best thing that could happen to me."

Many Japanese students work very hard in school.

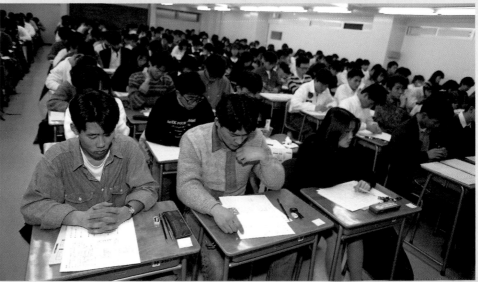

Readers' thoughts

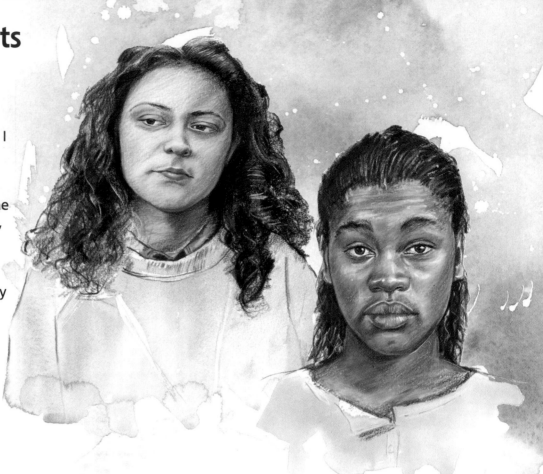

"I come from a Muslim family. I respect my parents and know what they expect of me. My family will arrange a suitable marriage for me when the time is right. I am prepared for this, but I also want to make sure that I have a career. I want to be a doctor. My parents are really pleased about this – they couldn't be more proud. They were a little concerned about the social activities at school. At my school, learning and socializing go together. After my parents talked with a Muslim teacher, they understood this better."
Fatima

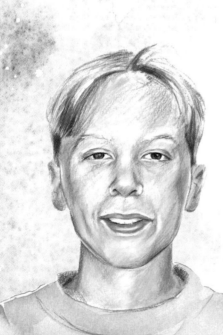

"My brother has this fixation about red. He has dyed every bit of clothing he owns and has painted his room all over – bright scarlet. His friends are all just as weird as he is. When they go around together, you can see other people moving away from them! I think it's all pretty silly. My brother looks kind of dangerous, but he's really a nice guy at heart. He goes around to see our grandma and grandpa every week. Their neighbors all expect him to steal from them, but it would never enter his head. I think it's a pity people judge him on his looks."
Peter

"Sometimes I think my parents don't care about me at all! They let me stay out late, and they don't seem to mind that I have friends they've never met. I talked to my mom about this, and she said that she wanted me to be able to express myself and learn about the world in my own way. Both she and Dad had very strict parents, and this made them unhappy. Don't get me wrong – I like going to parties and staying up late, but I also need somebody to talk to about stuff that I can't understand. I have made a really good friend who is older than me. He's telling me more than my parents ever have."
Lonnie

"There's a girl in our class who's hardly ever in school. She comes in the morning for attendance and then disappears after the first class. She's only 14 but looks at least four years older. One day I was coming back to school from a dentist appointment and saw her on a corner with a group of people, laughing and smoking. When I mentioned this to my friend, she said she'd seen her there too. It's where people hang out when they have nothing better to do. I don't want to tell on her, but she seems to be wasting her life. She'll never go anywhere at this rate."
Ava

"When I was 10, my parents told me I was adopted. That was quite a bombshell, I can tell you. I can't understand why they waited all that time before telling me. Maybe they thought I wouldn't be able to cope. I don't know. I was really upset to begin with. But when I thought about my friends' parents, I gradually came to admit that mine had usually treated me fairly. They were no nicer and no meaner to me than if I'd been their own child. And I can't ask for any more than that. I do wish they'd told me earlier, though."
Greg

"I've been going out with this nice girl, but recently she's become really clingy and possessive. I can't go anywhere or do anything without her wanting to come along, and it's really getting me down. I like her a lot but don't want her around all day. When I tell her gently and tactfully that I need some space, she takes it badly and thinks I don't like her anymore. Dealing with other people's feelings is the hardest thing I've ever had to do in my life."
Dominic

"I sometimes wonder if it's worth bothering. I try hard, but I never seem to be the best at anything I do. My best friend is near the top of our class and on every team there is. I'm average, and only once did I get to be a reserve on the football team. My dad says there's just a lot of bright kids in my class, and that's why I don't think I'm doing well. He says if I were in another class, I'd be near the top for sure. I guess that makes me feel a little better about it. Another thing that helps a lot is that I've got two kid brothers who look up to me and think I'm great. They give my ego a boost!"
Brett

You and the community

As you grow up, your sense of the world grows. It begins to expand past your home and your school to include your community, your country, and the world.

As you become more aware of the world around you, you'll discover things you like and things you don't. Many young people feel passionate about social issues and want to change the world. They care about poverty, sickness, war, and injustice, and want to fight them.

Many young people today are especially concerned about the environment: the destruction of the rain forest, the growing hole in the planet's protective ozone layer, air and water pollution, and the amount of garbage we produce. Others are moved by the plight of the homeless, the proliferation of drugs and gangs, or the need for AIDS research. Most young people are eager to devote time and energy to causes they believe in.

Stand up for a cause you believe in.

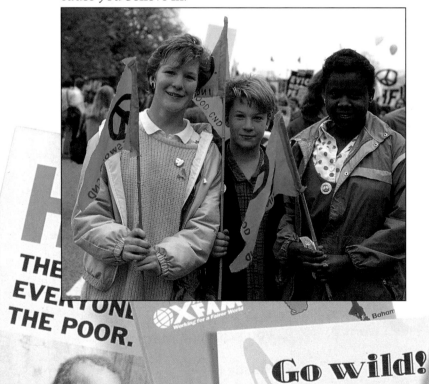

Local effort

When you look around your community, you're bound to find ways to make life better for people. For example, you could visit old or sick people. You could work with the physically handicapped in a hospital. You could volunteer to help in a church or community day-care center. You might organize a community cleanup. You and your friends could make an open space or park a nicer place to walk. You might learn CPR or first aid. The list of skills needed in a community is almost endless.

Don't forget politics. Living in a democracy gives you the opportunity to get involved in political discussion and campaigns. You may not be old enough to vote yet, but you're certainly old enough to stuff envelopes, make phone calls, and spread the word about a candidate who excites you.

Being active in your community can be rewarding. The more you put into your community, the more you will get out of it. You'll have a chance to meet and mix with people you might never have met. This may give you new experiences and different views on life. You'll find out how your community works too.

Find out about yourself

Work in the community also helps you discover your own talents. Sometimes community work can lead to a full-time career when you leave

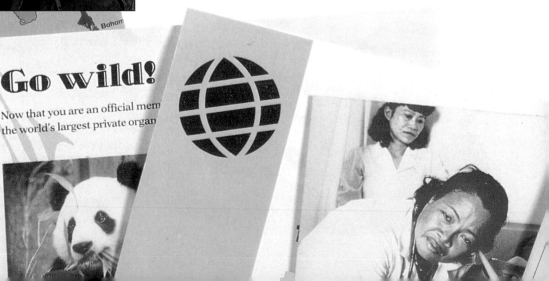

You can help make someone else's life easier and happier.

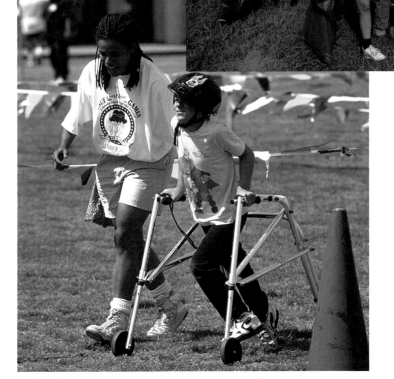

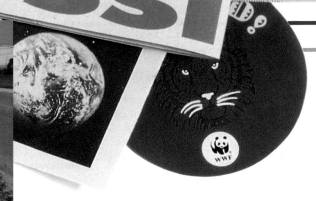

Keeping the earth clean is good for the environment.

school. For example, you may realize that you are good at raising money for organizations. This is a special talent. You need to be outgoing and trustworthy in order to persuade people to give you money for a cause.

You may discover that you are happiest working directly with disadvantaged people. Perhaps you're good with children, or you may find you are sympathetic and understanding with older people.

Global issues

Satellites beam powerful images of the world into our homes. When you see pictures of war, famine, or natural disasters on your television set, you may feel a little frustrated and powerless. What can you do about it?

Organizations such as Amnesty International, CARE, Greenpeace, the Red Cross, Save the Children, and the World Wildlife Fund are waiting for you to help. What cause interests you the most? A political cause? Humanitarian aid? Environmental concern? You can help by raising money for the cause that you care most deeply about. Some organizations may even have a group at the local level that you can join.

When you join a group and start working for a cause that you believe in, you gain too. You will have the opportunity to meet people – many with the same interests as yourself – as well as to learn more about the issue. The better informed you are, the more useful you'll be to your cause. You'll be able to explain its aims to other people and widen its impact on society.

Don't give up

Don't forget, water will wear away stone. Sometimes it takes a lifetime or longer to bring about change. When you're young, it's easy to feel frustrated with delays or lack of action. However, our commitment to making the world a better place must continue. And who knows what you might achieve.

NAMES, ADDRESSES, AND WEB SITES OF ORGANIZATIONS

Amnesty International	**Care**	**Greenpeace International**	**Red Cross**
322 Eighth Avenue	151 Ellis Street, NE	704 H Street, NW	431 18th Street, NW
New York, NY 10001	Atlanta, GA 30303-2440	Washington, DC 20001	Washington, DC 20006
www.amnesty.org	www.care.org	www.greenpeace.org	www.redcross.org

Look in your phone book to see if there are local chapters of these or other organizations you may be interested in helping.

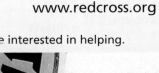

Acknowledgments

The publishers would like to thank the following for permission to use photographs in this book:

Adams Picture Library 20;
Collections 20, 22/23, 24/25, 32, 49;
David Hoffman Photolibrary 10/11, 34;
Format 56;
© Getty Images 28, 34;
Network Photographers 34;
© Tony Freeman, PhotoEdit 57;
© Michael Newman, PhotoEdit 17;
David Hoffman Photolibrary 10/11, 34;
National Slidebank 35;
Picturepoint Ltd. 18/19;
Rex Features 20/21;
Sally and Richard Greenhill 10, 20, 21, 42, 46, 49, 54;
Science Photo Library 33;
© Elizabeth Crews, The Image Works 12;
© Bob Daemmrich, The Image Works 34, 57;
The Metropolitan Police Service New Scotland Yard 36/37

Cover photos: © SuperStock; © Arthur Tilley, Getty Images; © Merritt A. Vincent, PhotoEdit; © Bonnie Kamin, PhotoEdit

The publishers would also like to give special thanks to everyone who acted as photographic models, and to Tisha for assistance with makeup.